PRAISE FOR
Dr. Ro's Ten Secrets to Livin' Healthy

"Praise to Dr. Ro for offering us such a clear process for caring for our body temples. We need to know what works and what doesn't, what to do and how we must do it to get results. *Dr. Ro's Ten Secrets* is cl_____ and practical. Read it. _____ well!"

  —Iyanla Vanzant, bests_____

"Dr. Ro's 'ten secrets to _____ _____. They are science-based a____ _____rally relevant."

  —David Satcher, M.D., 16th U.S. Surgeon General

"A valuable and inspirational book on how to eat and exercise. If African American women use this book as a guide, it will bring about a complete revolution in the health and well-being of the black community. Follow her advice, cook a few of her recipes, and see for yourself."

  —Floyd J. Malveaux, M.D., Ph.D.,
  Executive Director of the Merck
  Childhood Asthma Network

"Minorities are more likely than whites to have health problems, including obesity. Clearly we must take our health matters into our own hands. We desperately need to know Dr. Ro's ten secrets, and *use* them!"

  —Congressman Jesse L. Jackson Jr.

"Dr. Ro's book is written to create a healthy mind-set which will produce healthy choices by the reader. It is insightful, life-changing and I couldn't put it down! As a cancer conquerer I strongly recommend it to anyone who is serious about livin' healthy. This book is going to change lives!" —Les Brown, author of *Live Your Dreams*

"This book will help you to move on, move up, and move ahead in living the best and healthiest life possible. Read it, reread it, and tell your friends and family. Once you do, livin' the good life will be a secret no more." —Malik Yoba, actor

"Dr. Ro has produced a seminal work which provides highly accurate nutrition information in a very readable format. It reads almost like a novel."
—Allan A. Johnson, Ph.D., L.N., Professor and Chairman, Department of Nutritional Sciences, Howard University

"Dr. Ro is the bomb! I highly recommend *Dr. Ro's Ten Secrets to Livin' Healthy*. It will help you physically, mentally, and spiritually!"
—Willie Jolley, author of *A Setback Is a Setup for a Comeback* and *It Only Takes a Minute to Change Your Life*

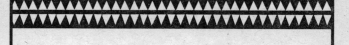

Dr.Ro's
Ten
Secrets to
Livin' Healthy

**America's Most Renowned
African American Nutritionist
Shows You How to Look Great,
Feel Better, and Live Longer
by Eating Right**

Rovenia M. Brock, Ph.D.

BANTAM BOOKS

DR. RO'S TEN SECRETS TO LIVIN' HEALTHY
A Bantam Book

PUBLISHING HISTORY
Bantam hardcover edition published January 2004
Bantam trade paperback edition / January 2005
Bantam mass market edition / January 2008

Published by Bantam Dell
A Division of Random House, Inc.
New York, New York

Book design by Virginia Norey

Library of Congress Catalog Card Number: 2003056272

ISBN 978-0-553-58558-2

Manufactured in the United States of America
Published simultaneously in Canada

OPM 10 9 8 7 6 5 4 3 2

A woman is free if she prizes her own individuality, creates her own destiny, and puts no boundaries on her hopes for tomorrow.

▼▼▼▼

For Yvette —
Use this work to grow —
Stretch — & be fabulous!

xox
— DR. R

For Larvenia and Rosetta, who loved me more than I thought humanly possible. For my husband, Murray, who today picks up where they left off. And for the multitude of sisters who await the opportunity to give themselves permission and who need the motivation to put their lives in order; use this work to take the first steps of your journey.

Contents

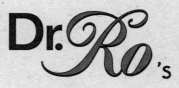

Ten
Secrets to
Livin' Healthy

Secret 1

To Change Your Life,
You Have to Change Your Mind

 My mother, Larvenia Brock, who got pregnant with me, her only child, when she was 44 years old, died from stomach cancer when I was 9. She was diagnosed with the deadly disease the same year I was born.

Larvenia had a very independent, entrepreneurial spirit—she owned a successful cab company in Washington, D.C., which she ran during the week, and operated a thriving juke joint on weekends—but she couldn't translate her business smarts into smart health choices. Though my mother in her younger days was a shapely bombshell with an hourglass figure, she didn't lose her pregnancy weight after my birth and remained heavy throughout my childhood. To add insult to injury, healthy eating wasn't on her radar screen. Believe me, you rarely get stomach cancer unless something is really wrong with your diet. And something was definitely wrong with my mother's diet. Larvenia never met a steak she didn't like; she ate chitlins on holidays and downed pig feet and whiskey on weekends at the juke joint. Though vegetables were plentiful in our house, they were usually prepared with lard or fatback and either deep-fried or slow-cooked until all the nutrients leached out.

That diet finally caught up with my mother, and she became very sick. The overweight powerhouse I had known for my first nine years ended up confined to bed, a tiny, shrunken shell of her former self. During her final days she was unable to keep down even a forkful of watermelon, which had been one of her favorites. Her best friend, Rosetta Lewis, would send me off for it, saying, "Run to the store as fast as your little legs will carry you." I did, thinking if I could just make it to Safeway, get my mom's watermelon, and race back without delay, I could somehow stop the bandit that was robbing me of my precious mother. I was wrong. Even the love and unyielding dedication of a 9-year-old could not stop the inevitable. Finally, the person I depended on for everything, even life itself, died. The devastation of that blow crippled my spirit.

On her deathbed, Larvenia left instructions for Rosetta to raise me, with the assistance of my extended family, to adulthood. Rosetta was a wonderful second mother to me, but unfortunately her health choices weren't any better than Larvenia's had been. She overate on a regular basis. She had lived through the Depression, so throwing away food was unthinkable. A native of Rocky Mount, North Carolina, Rosetta was accustomed to eating standard southern fare: greens seasoned with fatback, pig feet, potato salad, chitlins, pork chops, and anything smothered in rich gravy, including crispy fried chicken and rabbit. Over the years, I watched Rosetta battle heart disease, high blood pressure, and breast cancer—all illnesses that probably could have been prevented, or at least delayed or lessened, had she chosen a healthier lifestyle. Despite the duration and variety of her ailments, Rosetta lived to be 86, so I got to have her with me until 1996. Some of you might ask, "What's wrong with that? She lived a long life, right?" Well, yes, she did, but it certainly was a hard one. Her kidneys had failed, her heart problems weakened her, and eight years before she died she suffered a stroke that left her paralyzed on her left side. That she had a long life is true. But was her quality of life what it could have been? I think not.

A Product of the Environment

By now I have learned an enormous amount about food and physical activity and their relationship to health, but when I was growing up I had no concept of a healthy diet. I ate what my family ate: country ham and fried salt fish (sodium count through the roof), scrapple, fried potatoes and onions, fried apples, hoecake (a corn bread of white cornmeal and water cooked on top of the stove in a skillet), and my grandma's "stand-up-straight" coffee (we called it that because it was so strong it could almost stand on its own). And that was just for breakfast! Sure, I flirted briefly with being what a friend and I thought of as "vegetarian" when we were in high school, but that was because it was a fad, not a choice I made in the interest of health. For lunch my friend and I would bring cans of tuna and shrimp and make salads. Our food looked more interesting and appealing than the cafeteria's offerings, and we became the cool kids, setting the lunchtime style for the rest of the student body.

Even that casual flirtation with a different way of eating didn't last long, because along with my mother's strong spirit, I also inherited her love of steak and fried foods. Despite the fact that my mother's early death had shown me there is a connection between healthy eating and a healthy life, I developed an addiction to the steak and cheese subs from Trio's. If you've never had a steak and cheese (excuse me, Philly folk, but in D.C. we call 'em steak and cheese, not cheese steaks) from Trio's, a fixture in Washington, D.C.'s restaurant world, you haven't really lived. There's so much seasoned meat on this sandwich, it's as if a cow wandered onto a sub roll and fell apart. All kidding aside, there must be 18 ounces of meat on one-half of the sub, not to mention the slices of provolone cheese that complete the sandwich. But because I'd always been a fairly trim person, I thought I could eat anything I wanted without paying the price of weight gain. And until I turned 26, I did. I weighed somewhere around 99 pounds.

Actually, like a lot of black women, in my teens and twenties I worried not about being too fat but about being too skinny. When you keep hearing how you need to put a little meat on your bones and get yourself some curves, it gets to you. And the truth was, I really was too thin. Although I was a grown woman, I had a childlike body, and I figured surely the brothas would be more attracted to me if I looked more like a woman. So when I was in my mid-20s, even though I was now a practicing nutritionist in hospitals and nursing homes with a lot of knowledge about what a healthy diet should be, I began a program of intentionally overeating—and you better believe it wasn't fruits and vegetables, soy, and whole grains I was gobbling down. No, it was those steak and cheese subs I mentioned earlier, mammoth amounts of ice cream, and all kinds of junk food. I made sure to go to bed on a full stomach every night, and I was eating like this all in the interest of gaining the kind of weight that would make me more desirable. Needless to say, my strategy worked, and I gained plenty of weight—about 30 pounds in all. I thought I looked great, and there were plenty of friends and relatives congratulating me on my new curves.

But eventually, after about four or five years of intentional overeating, life had its way with me. One day I looked at myself in a mirror and in shock wondered aloud, "Who the hell is that following me back there?" It happened while I was out shopping with a friend. As shocked as I was, however, I didn't do anything about it. In fact, things were about to get worse.

The very next year, 1987, when I was 31, I quit my job to enter graduate school in nutrition. It was a really exciting time for me, because not only was I studying for an advanced degree, but I also began my television career, signing on to serve as the nutrition correspondent for a newsmagazine show on Howard University's PBS station. This was the beginning of many years of work on television and radio, which included stints for the Howard PBS affiliate and eventually for Black Entertainment Television (BET), where I had various gigs as health correspondent, general assignment reporter, and medical correspondent. Later I also worked for the University of the District of Columbia, hosting both TV and radio shows. There was even a year when I was on TV and radio for UDC *and* doing a nutrition news segment for an NBC affiliate.

Needless to say, I seemed to be on the move every minute of the day during those insanely busy years, so I was always grabbing food on the run, snacking every chance I got, eating larger amounts of food more often. With time being such a precious commodity, I developed the habit of scarfing down poorly planned meals of fast food to survive. Although it was a contradiction to be pursuing an education in nutrition while ignoring the information that I was gaining in my own life, that's exactly what I did during all my years of graduate school.

By age 34, I felt like I had finally arrived. I had completed my master's degree in nutrition and broadcast journalism, and I was now a health correspondent on a national news show that aired once a week on Black Entertainment Television. Life was good. But even while I was gaining greater success in my television career, I kept my education goals center stage and began working on a doctorate. As life got ever busier and crazier, I was eating myself into two dress sizes larger than I had ever been in my life.

But even then I kept getting the "you look good with a little weight on your bones" comments. Friends and family applauded the extra weight. So I listened to them, lied to myself that it was okay, and gradually ate myself into a size 8. This may not sound so big to you, but a size 8 body on a frame that's supposed to fit into a size 4 is not a pretty sight. By age 37, I was an overweight nutritionist and television personality. My career was still going well, but my spirits were low, because I knew my life had spun out of control. There I was on television telling people how to eat, but I wasn't following my own advice, and anyone could tell that just from looking at me. The hypocrisy began to consume me. I had to do something about it.

Making the Lifestyle-Diet Connection

Watching the two most important women in my life suffer from diseases that were at least partly diet-related should've scared me straight long before then. And on some level this did happen, inspiring my choice of a career, even though I wasn't putting what I learned in my nutrition classes and preached on my television shows into practice. It amazes me now to think about how I continued to live such an unhealthy lifestyle despite what I knew. Not only did I have my mother and Rosetta as examples, but even before my mother got sick I was aware that black people had all kinds of health problems because of what they ate. I remember that I first made a connection between health and diet in elementary school, when my friend Bryant's dad had to have his legs "cut off"—because of "di-a-bee-tes," Bryant said. I asked my mother why this was happening to him, and her explanation was that people who had "a touch of sugar" had to watch what they ate.

Gradually I realized that having a "touch of sugar" described practically everyone in my family and my community. What I began to notice as time marched on was that like Bryant's dad, people did not in fact watch what they ate, and many of their health problems were the result.

My understanding of the role of food in health and disease increased during frequent trips to the hospital with my mother. It was during those years that I first realized I was interested in nutrition. This was thanks to Ruby Cavanaugh, the dietitian who counseled patients at the hospital about their food habits. Ruby, who was a friend of my mother's, used to take me to her office while my mother was being seen by her doctors. Spending time in her office, I first saw up close and on a rather personal level what important work this could be. I was very young, only 9 years of age, but even I could see that "Mrs. Cavanaugh" had something to do with making people feel better through food.

By the time I was old enough to go to college, I knew I wanted to study nutrition as a profession, because my family and my community needed help. The hit list of diseases and conditions that plague us— hypertension, heart disease, obesity, diabetes, cancer— were in my family and all around me. During college I started to make more of a connection between what I was learning in my textbooks and the lifestyle choices people made that led to poor health. And when I did two internships at Howard University Hospital, I saw hundreds of people whose experience mirrored what was going on with my family and in the community. I realized that many diseases these people suffered from began with or were made worse by what they ate.

By the way, it was Ruby Cavanaugh—the same dietitian in whose office I spent so much time almost 20 years earlier, when my mother was in the hospital—who became my teacher when I began my internship in nutrition. So it's in part thanks to her that I now preach the gospel of nutrition and the importance of a healthy lifestyle. I do it because of Larvenia and Rosetta. I do it because of my community, my fellow black people. I do it because I want you, sista-friends, to make the changes necessary to live healthy, full, productive lives. And I do it for myself, too. But I didn't start on my own path to health until years after I'd been preaching it to others.

Taking My First Steps

In order to lose all the unhealthy weight I'd gained by age 37, I first had to make a mental commitment to change. That's everybody's first step, and everyone has a different motivation for doing it, usually some kind of wake-up call having to do with either the way they feel or the way they look. I have to admit that at first my own motivation was mainly vanity. I'd been aware for quite some time that I didn't look as if I was practicing what I was preaching, but what really jump-started my commitment to change—and I'm sure you'll recognize this kind of incentive for weight loss—was a big event that was suddenly on the horizon. I was invited to a formal affair where I would be given the first ever Rovenia Brock Excellence in

Journalism Award by Swing Phi Swing Social Fellowship, a women's sorority of sorts to which I had belonged since college. For this very swanky affair I wanted to look my best. Showing up without all curves tightly tucked into place, arms buffed and toned, and thighs and butt slimmed simply would not do. What would people think?

Lucky for me, I was in the position of being able to use what I did at work to get to work on myself. I was at that time hosting my first cable television show in Washington, D.C., *At Your Service*, which was a government-funded consumer affairs television show that gave me free rein to do just about anything I wanted, as long as I helped someone in my audience while I did it. It occurred to me that I could focus my show for the next several months on my own weight loss diet and exercise regimen, inviting my viewers to join me in learning a healthier way of life. Each week I would give them nutrition pointers, heart-healthy recipes, tips on exercise, and so on. If they could eat the way I encouraged them to eat, and follow my exercise routine, we'd all have a win-win scenario. So I started by working out with a personal trainer on the air. The cameras followed us to the YMCA, where we worked out, combining strength training with aerobics. We began with two days a week; then as things progressed we stuffed three and sometimes four days a week into both our busy schedules.

This turned out to be a great plan. Not only was I sticking to my commitment, but I was inspiring members of my audience to make a commitment to getting healthy, too. The support I got from them was tremendous, and I surely needed it. I received letters, phone calls, and many requests on the street—in the grocery store, in line at the bank, and in restaurants—to help women shed their unwanted pounds. I was the nutritionist they saw as having it all together, the expert who could help them by serving as their example. The show was a success, and so, after several months, was I. When I walked up to the dais to receive my journalism award at the Swing Phi Swing event, I looked exactly the way I had hoped I would.

As I think back now on my zeal for fitness at that time, I realize that I was pumped up to do the right thing for all of the wrong reasons. That's probably why my weight loss didn't last. Within six months of that gala affair, I had stopped working out with the trainer, I did nothing on my own, and—you guessed it—I'd ballooned again. I was having exactly the same experience most dieters have: a brief period of inspiration and terrific results, followed by a return to the pre-diet weight, and eventually even more pounds than I had before I started. In the months that followed I'd have short periods of trying to get back to an exercise routine, but they never lasted, and I continued to struggle with my eating habits, too. Since I'd spent so many years eating whatever I wanted, whenever I wanted, and in any amount, I found it hard to break the old habits. My addiction to the steak subs at Trio's was no exception. In fact, during the next couple of years I frequently took visiting friends there at 2 A.M. after getting off work.

By 1996 I not only had my own local cable television show, *At Your Service with Dr. Rovenia Brock*, but also a daily, hour-long radio show bearing the same name. Though my schedule was absolutely insane, I had finally finished my Ph.D., and my work in TV and radio had taken a giant leap, so I was now on my way to doing what I had always wanted to do—making a full-time career of giving the public information about how to take better care of themselves. The problem was, once again I wasn't taking my own advice, and the result was that I was now heavier than I'd ever been— a size 10.

So two years after my first experience with a personal trainer, I did another self-evaluation and decided for the second time that I would make myself into an on-air experiment in healthy living. In search of yet another savior, I wandered into the fitness center near my office and found just the person I was looking for. This time it would be Megan who'd whip me into shape, and we'd be doing our work for the benefit of my radio audience. Each week I informed my radio show listeners of my progress and talked to them about the exercise routines I was following, the diet I put myself on, and the health benefits I enjoyed as a result. They loved it. Many of them called and wrote to tell us that they were rooting for me and that they would step up to the proverbial plate themselves. In the course of three months I lost several inches off my waist, hips, and thighs; got fit enough that I could climb several flights of stairs without feeling winded; and by the end of six months had lost 15 pounds and still more inches. Fifteen pounds may not sound like much, but it added up to a lot of inches, because thanks to all the weight training my fat was being replaced by muscle, which weighs a lot more than fat but takes up less space and looks a lot better! During this time I also adopted a cute little cocker spaniel, Destinye, who became my muse for long walks and jogging in the park. She gave me no choice but to get my butt out of bed each morning at six to let her do her business. Because I had to walk Destinye (who loves a good run) I was forced to work some exercise into my day even when I didn't want to. About three months of this and it became second nature. Walking was now a part of me.

Unfortunately, the weight didn't stay lost this time, either. Although I kept up my walking, I also kept up my eating—and then some. My quick morning and evening walks with Destinye weren't nearly enough to counteract my unhealthy eating habits, but I couldn't seem to change my diet, and without Megan to encourage me, I'd stopped my gym workouts, too. So I gained back much of what I had lost.

Fast-forward another three years to the first season of *Heart & Soul* on Black Entertainment Television. This was yet another huge career leap for me, because for the first time I was serving as a co-host on a national television show. The pressure was really on, too, because not only was this a much bigger deal than anything I'd worked on before, but it had a younger, hipper demographic, and suddenly, at the age of 43 and at a size 8, three sizes larger than what I am now, I was expected to shoehorn myself into the show's typical funky, tight, skimpy wardrobe. Mocha, my co-host, was a buff beauty who was built like a brick house. Sitting next to her on the set was what really provided me with the motivation to once again get my butt (pun intended) in gear. Also, just in case I hadn't gotten the point myself, a few close friends had dutifully mentioned something that was already dawning on me: The last thing anyone wants to see on TV is an overweight nutritionist telling you how you should eat. I decided that if I couldn't practice what I was preaching, I might as well get out of the business.

It is no accident that today I dole out lots of advice about how to cut calories and that one of the suggestions I make most often is to always leave food on your plate. Sistas, I've tried it myself, so I *know* it works. I began by making this behavioral change at Trio's, eating only half of my favorite steak and cheese. Don't get me wrong—I still wanted the whole thing, but I had to start someplace. Did I stop going to Trio's altogether? I won't lie—that steak and cheese sub called to me like Richard Pryor's crack pipe in the corner. But I fought the temptation. Having succeeded at Trio's, I expanded my plan, cutting portions by leaving some food on my plate at all my meals, no matter what or where I was eating. I filled up on water before eating, concentrated on the conversation instead of the food during meals, and in general tried to focus more on the incredible rush I got from my job rather than on my enjoyment of food.

Did my aunts and cousins keep encouraging me to "eat up" at Thanksgiving and family meals? Damn skippy they did, but I had a career to protect, so I did what I had to do. And while I continued to make changes in my eating habits, I also knew I had to stop fooling myself and get serious about working out again. One night around this time I was attending a concert during the Congressional Black Caucus Foundation's Annual Legislative Conference and saw a woman I couldn't stop staring at. It was her arms that grabbed my attention. She looked entirely feminine, but she had beautifully defined arms—so striking that I approached her and asked if she worked out, because I wanted to know what her secret was. With a pleasant nod she confirmed that she did work out; in fact, she trained people for a living. I struck a deal with her that if she could help me get into shape, she'd give me a discount on her regular rates and I'd refer her to everyone I knew.

Patricia came to my home to do an evaluation of me so that she could determine where we should start. About a year earlier I had broken an ankle in two places, so I was nervous about reinjuring myself while working out. After her baseline evaluation, using my treadmill, she saw exactly how out of shape I was. Not only was I out of shape in terms of my cardiovascular fitness, but I wanted to drop at least two dress sizes to get to where I should be for my small frame. Patricia assured me that together we could get there but warned that I had a lot of work in front of me. Just as alarming, for the first time I wasn't allowed to use my status as a minor celebrity on a TV or radio show to get a trainer. No, this time I had to pay out of my own pocket. Even though I was getting a discount, it was still going to cost what seemed like a lot of money to me. For someone who'd never paid for that kind of thing before, this was a colossal step. Surely, I'd happily spend a few hundred dollars at a time on a new dress or shoes, but blow money on a trainer? No way. I had to be honest with myself, though. If I was serious about making a lasting change in my approach to good health, I needed the motivation that Patricia could give me. I decided to save some of the money I spent on suits and clothes for the camera and put it toward a much more permanent way of looking good. Finally I was putting my money where my mouth was—on my own good health. I thought of the money I spent on Patricia as an investment in my career, my looks, and my life.

We began walking, even during the coldest winter days. We would walk for half an hour, then do strength-training exercises for the following half hour. We walked using the treadmill or in the park. Up hills, down hills, across rugged terrain—it didn't matter to Pat. She was on a mission to speed up my metabolism. In addition to the half-hour workouts we did on our walking days, we did hour-long strength-training workouts two days a week, then progressed to three days a week. The walking we did was for fat burning and cardiovascular conditioning, and the strength training, which we did with free weights (dumbbells), was for muscle building and toning. Most days her routines were grueling. She had me doing crunches, inverted crunches, leg lifts, side leg lifts, triceps kickbacks, and triceps dips to make those sagging granny arms disappear. Besides the dumbbells, we used anything in or around the house for equipment, from the side of the bathtub for triceps exercises to the front steps for cardiovascular work.

I had to admit there were days when I wanted to

quit, but Patricia, who had become my confidante and my friend as well as my trainer, wouldn't hear of my failing. As far as she was concerned, that would mean that she had failed, and she wasn't willing to consider failure as an option—for either her or me. For the third time I began to see the inches disappearing from all over my body, even as my biceps and triceps muscles were developing and becoming newly visible now that the fat wasn't covering them up. I had been through this process enough times, finally, to understand that the only way to achieve lasting effects on my health and on my appearance was through working out. Though I'd gotten the food issues under control some time before, it had taken me a while to come to grips with the fact that the moment I slowed down my activity level, the weight was sure to come back, even if my eating habits remained sound. And that weight was going to come to rest on my thighs and hips and all the other parts of my body—and on my spirit as well. Eventually I felt psyched enough to begin working out on my own. Patricia remained my friend but was no longer my trainer. And this time I was able to *keep* myself motivated.

Even on those days when I wanted nothing more than to stay under the covers for an extra hour of shut-eye, I hauled my butt out of bed and, with Destinye in tow, hit the pavement. The experts say it takes only three weeks to form a habit. According to Dr. Louis Aronne, an obesity specialist at New York–Presbyterian Hospital, doing anything repeatedly for three weeks—even a fitness regimen—triggers habit formation in our systems. Dr. Aronne says there are several stages to successfully forming a habit: pre-contemplation (I thought about my weight gain predicament), contemplation (I wanted to do something about it), preparation (I hired a trainer to help me stay motivated to make a positive change), action (I actually worked out and changed my diet and eating habits), maintenance (I kept up my end of the bargain for four to six months at a time), and finally, alas, backsliding. Remember, I enlisted the help of a trainer three different times to lose the same 15 pounds, so to say I know something about backsliding is an understatement. But I knew enough by now not to give up, to just make myself start over again, because every day is a new day. The fact that I have continued my 6 A.M. workouts and my calorie-cutting tactics (for the most part, anyway) is a testament to the effectiveness of habit formation. After getting into a routine for at least three weeks, it had finally once again become a part of me. Only this time it was real.

I persevered with my new regimen, because week after week I'd watch the tapes of myself on *Heart & Soul* and think, "That extra 20 pounds has got to go!" The 20 pounds I was trying to get rid of, on top of the 20 pounds TV adds to your face—and the rest of you—really made me look fatter than anyone who called herself a nutritionist should be.

As I kept on keeping on, I didn't tell anyone what I was doing. I had done that too often before. So this time I just tried to work quietly on myself and hoped that eventually people would notice without my having to call attention to the results. Notice they did! My public encouraged me to stay in the fight, both for my sake and for theirs. Once again sistas like you called, e-mailed, wrote letters, and stopped me on the street, on a national ten-city tour I was doing, the Tampax Total You Tour, to say I was an inspiration. That was reward and pressure all rolled into one!

Taking Your First Steps

Now we're all in this fight together. Armed with the right information and an ounce of discipline, we've got the right recipe for success. You may struggle a bit at first, too. Still, we have to understand that there's a link between our Saturday night drinking binges, our holiday chitlin meals, our church-on-Sunday fried chicken dinners, our cigarette-smoking obsessions, and the state of chronic ill health in which most of us find ourselves. In our high-tech society we'd like to believe that we can deal with the consequences of overconsumption immediately by getting a shot, taking a pill, or drinking a special potion. But it's not that simple. Just because you decide it's time for a change doesn't mean you'll be able to make it happen overnight.

Melinda's Story: ✦ Melinda Jefferson, a fan of *Heart & Soul*, understands this. She's a 24-year-old woman who, as she says, was always "a heavyset child." Her twin sister, Lucinda, was heavy, too. As is often the case in the black community, family members didn't see anything wrong with the girls' excessive weight; in fact, many of these relatives were overweight as well. Both girls spent much of their childhood eating fatty foods with hardly a thought about what these foods might be doing to their health. In fact, nobody ever gave a thought to how their diets might be affecting the girls' future health, even though Melinda's mother, several aunts, and two grandparents suffered from diabetes and high blood pressure. "No one made the connection to dietary habits, or between being sedentary and being sick," Melinda says now.

Identifying the Problem: ✦ Melinda's weight, when it was thought about as a problem at all, was only an issue of dress size. Melinda's twin, Lucinda, had lost 50 pounds in high school because she didn't want to be fat at her prom. But Melinda didn't go to her prom, so she didn't even think about losing weight. Then, during college, she not only gained the infamous freshman 15, but kept on accumulating pounds throughout her school years. "My joints hurt," she says. "I was out of breath just walking to the mailbox. I couldn't find attractive clothes, and I was uncomfortable in cars. Flying was almost out of the question." Still, she didn't see the link between her weight and her health.

Then Lucinda got pregnant. Seeing her twin eat for two, Melinda thought, "If she can eat, so can I." Sadly, Melinda's weight ballooned to a whopping 300 pounds.

One afternoon shortly after her niece's birth, Melinda experienced severe chest pains. The pains turned out not to be anything serious, but when she overheard the folks in the emergency room talking about her weight and expressing surprise that she hadn't had some sort of serious health issue before then, she became frightened by the prospect of what could happen.

It was at this point that Melinda recognized she had to make some changes. "I was determined that my weight had gone up as much as I could stand. I kept thinking that if I could just eat less food, I'd lose the weight. But I kept gaining. I'd skip breakfast, have a big fast-food lunch, then skip dinner," she says. Then, late at night, Melinda, starving, would raid the refrigerator and the kitchen pantry. "I thought I was eating less—and during the day I was. But the calories I ate for lunch were mostly all fat calories, and I didn't count the after-dinner calories from my nightly binges." Soon she was tipping the scales at 347 pounds. "I was frustrated and depressed. I wanted to lose weight, but what I was doing wasn't working."

Then, when Lucinda's daughter was a year old, she started trying to lose the weight she'd gained during her pregnancy, and she began to make some headway in the struggle. Meanwhile, an overweight family friend, having recently been diagnosed with diabetes, had also embarked on the weight loss path. Seeing the commitment of these two women, Melinda was inspired to try to tackle her own weight problems. So two years ago she made the decision to change her lifestyle in a radical way.

Creating a Plan: ✦ First, Melinda decided to reduce her fat intake by cutting out all fried foods, fast foods, and meats. It wasn't easy at first. "I felt like I was starving all day long," she says. "And I missed my pork chops and my Whoppers with Cheese something terrible!"

But she'd heard my *Heart & Soul* mantra to drink a minimum of eight 8-ounce glasses of water a day, so she committed to drinking that 64 ounces every day. The water took some of the edge off her hunger by filling her up and gave her sluggish metabolism a boost.

Next she decided that she needed to start doing some exercise. So she waded through feelings of inadequacy and embarrassment as she made her way to the gym to work out. "Everybody else there seemed to be thin and already in shape. I was the only whale in that place," she jokes now. "I just knew they were all talking about me behind my back."

Determined, Melinda started on Nautilus machines, 30 minutes at a time, every day. She had heard my reports on *Heart & Soul* that weight training not only strengthened bones but also burned calories. But Melinda wasn't quite prepared for what she would learn about herself. "Surprisingly, working out was actually harder than cutting back on the food," she says. "I was so out of shape. I had never really been active before then, not even as a child, and I hated every minute of it in the beginning. I watched the clock so I could hop off the equipment the second my 30 minutes were done." Within a month, however, she was extending her gym visits beyond that half hour; some days she didn't even realize how much time had passed. She just knew she was starting to feel better about herself.

Watching *Heart & Soul*, Melinda had also learned that walking is a good way to get an easy workout, particularly if you're not an athlete. Interestingly enough, a workout buddy at the gym suggested she start walking, so Melinda switched from the Nautilus and put on her walking shoes, traveling a mile a day. For a while she was joined on these treks by the two women who had first inspired her to lose weight, but then Melinda got ambitious and decided to switch from walking to jogging, and because her sister and friend wanted to stick with walking she was now on her own. "The hardest part about jogging was figuring out how to breathe properly to maintain my stamina," she says. So she turned to a high school cross-country coach for tips. Even then, she could barely jog a mile. But she strapped on her Walkman and "put one foot in front of the other. Each day I ran at least one additional block," she says. Now Melinda runs three miles a day, and Lucinda walks at least one. She and her sister each pay a $20 penalty if either of them backslides.

Was it easy to do? Hardly. Melinda is quick to admit she has driven to late-night fast-food joints on more than one occasion, then eaten her taboo booty in secret in her car, praying no one would look through her window and catch her. And there are days when she would've preferred a root canal to that three-mile run. But her results tell a real success story. She lost 10 pounds the first week, and though she knew it was mostly water, it kept her motivated enough to stick with the plan. A year after starting her quest for health, Melinda had lost 45 pounds. She'd replaced high-fat meals such as hamburger and ribs with baked chicken and tuna. And she'd started keeping a food log, because, as she puts it, "I'd be lost without it." To date, she has lot a total of 90 pounds. That's what I call coming a long way! Her journey from weighing in at more than 300 pounds is not over—she figures she still has another 97 pounds to go—but she has made the necessary adjustments to change her lifestyle. And she's so thrilled with the results that she's finding it easier and easier to stick to her commitment.

Battling Denial

Ever greater numbers of Americans, according to a report released by former U.S. Surgeon General David Satcher just before he left the Surgeon General's office in early 2002, are becoming overweight (defined as having a BMI of 25 or greater) and obese (a BMI of 30 or more). The report estimates that a staggering 61 percent of American adults currently meet the medical definition of overweight or obese, putting them at increased risk of heart disease, diabetes, stroke, arthritis, depression, and several forms of cancer. Each year, nearly 300,000 deaths can be attributed to this epidemic. Obesity rates have gone up 30 percent since the 1970s, and only one-third of U.S. adults meet recommendations for at least 30 minutes of exercise five days per week. The report attributes this hefty increase to poor diets and the sedentary lifestyles that have become synonymous with American culture.

These rates are even higher in the African American community. According to the third National Health and Nutrition Examination Survey (1988–1994), nearly 79 percent of black women in this country are overweight or obese, compared to less than 50 percent of white women.

Now, you may be one of those sistas who thinks, "That report doesn't apply to me. I'm nothing like Melinda; I don't weigh 300 pounds." You may think you've got your act together. As long as you can wiggle into that size 10 sundress every year when the mercury hits 80 degrees, you figure you're just fine. Well, you may be fine—for now. But as time marches on, girlfriend, you'll find it more difficult to maintain your shape, energy level, weight, and health. Looking good is virtually effortless at 18, when you're more likely to be physically active, but keeping that physique and that glow as you age requires a great deal more than an occasional liquid diet and regular trips to the hairstylist and a day spa.

Unless you develop a plan, one day you will look up and realize, like I did, that there's an extra person behind you and you're about 10 minutes away from calling your mama's doctor, because you both have the same weight-related problems. You may be used to seeing how obesity, heart disease, diabetes, and high blood pressure affect your mother, aunts, and older sisters as the years go by, but that does not have to be their fate. Nor does it have to be yours.

Rationalizing Yourself to Death

Will you need to adjust your attitude before you can start your personal journey to a healthy lifestyle? Yes. This is especially true if you're one of those sistas who tells herself one (or more!) of the following rationalizations:

❖ **Rationalization #1:** So what if those chitlins are a little fatty? Hot sauce and vinegar will burn it off, and they taste good.

❖ **Truth:** Chitterlings are definitely a fat-laden food, and nothing you put on top of them will make them less so. They may taste good, but they have very little nutritional value.

❖ **Rationalization #2:** That "thin is in" stuff is the white world's perpetuation of European ideals; we're supposed to have a little meat on our bones.

❖ **Truth:** You might hear this comment from your grandmother or great-aunt. One of my clients, Ann, was stick thin throughout her childhood and early adulthood, weighing in at about 110 pounds. By age 27, however, she'd started a sedentary job with long hours that left little time for physical activity. In addition to consuming fast food at nearly every meal, Ann ate the cookies, cakes, or doughnuts that always seemed to be in the office, and she gained 50 pounds in a two-year period. By the time she came to see me, she was still squeezing (barely) into her size 6 clothing, but she was unhappy with her potbelly, her jiggly thighs, and the rolls developing on her back. But every time Ann complained to her family about her weight gain, they said, "That's crazy talk. You needed to gain some weight, baby. Those curves look good on you. You ain't a white girl. Your body is different; you're *supposed* to be round." The truth is, your sista-body may be slightly different from a white woman's (more about this in

Secret 2), but this argument is just an excuse to lug around extra weight. You're not supposed to be overweight or obese, and you're certainly not supposed to be in ill health for the sake of a few extra curves.

✤ **Rationalization #3:** What does it matter if the potato salad and fried chicken dinner from last Sunday's church supper were loaded with fat? It was in church, and God can't be wrong. Right?

✤ **Truth:** C'mon, you're not going to blame God for your unhealthy eating choices, are you? God didn't fry that chicken in oil or use fatty mayonnaise in the potato salad. He didn't force you to eat it, either.

✤ **Rationalization #4:** I don't make enough money to lose weight. Only celebrities like Oprah and Janet Jackson, who have the money to hire a personal trainer, can afford to get in shape.

✤ **Truth:** African American women spend a small fortune on the things they want: acrylic nails, hair, makeup, clothes, and massages (61 percent more than their white counterparts). But if money really is an issue, and for some of you I know it is, you don't have to hire a personal trainer or join a gym to start being active. Walking in the park or the mall, roller-skating through the neighborhood, and jumping rope are free.

✤ **Rationalization #5:** I don't need to lose weight—girl, I look good in my clothes.

❖ **Truth:** If you keep buying a larger size to cover your ever-expanding girth, you'll look good in your casket, too.

❖ **Rationalization #6:** Beautiful women come in all shapes and sizes.
❖ **Truth:** They do. Healthy women, however, aren't carrying around 20, 30, or more pounds of excess weight. Health, unlike beauty, is *not* in the eye of the beholder.

❖ **Rationalization #7:** It's expensive to eat healthy.
❖ **Truth:** Go tell that to people who live on less money than you or I, yet manage to do so in a much more healthful way—thriving on diets of fruits, vegetables, grains, and little meat. Beans and brown rice cost pennies per serving, for example. But if you look at your grocery bill you'll see that meat is much more expensive than grains or fruits and vegetables, all of which are better for you. With proper planning, you can spend a minimum amount of money to achieve maximum nutritional health. I'm not asking you to become a vegetarian, but opting for meatless meals periodically will certainly give your health a boost. The fact is, many studies show that the more affluent people become, the worse their eating habits get. People who live in the Caribbean and in Africa eat much healthier diets, which do not include lots of fatty meat, and they weigh far less and suffer far fewer of the chronic diseases we have here in America.

What's Our Attitude Got to Do with It?

Sometimes these rationalizations lead to unhealthy bodies. When we're living in denial about our diet, our activity level, and our weight, we're likely to keep packing on extra pounds. And we're also likely to remain sedentary, not exercising our bodies—or our God-given right to rich, healthful lives. This, in turn, causes us to pack on (or keep on) extra pounds. It's a vicious cycle.

Does the way we think about our sista-bodies really affect our quality of life? In other words, what's our attitude got to do with it? In a word, everything! If you don't believe me, you can take a look at some of the research. Study upon study speaks volumes about how we think ourselves into bad health. One research survey of adults between 18 and 96 years old found that at 20 pounds more than their healthy weight, black respondents didn't think they had a weight problem at all. But 20 pounds more than your usual or healthy weight is enough to make you gasp for breath walking up and down stairs. And in some cases, 20 pounds is enough to be the difference between being healthy and not.

Interestingly, there are cultural factors that affect how we think about our bodies, and some of these may contribute to our weight problems. It's not just the notion that we don't want to look like one of those skinny, emaciated white women (see rationalization #2 above) because even when we do want to lose weight, according to University of Pennsylvania nutritional anthropologist Shiriki Kumanyika, Ph.D., we have a negative attitude about weight loss success stories if they come from women of other races. When we hear that Susie White Woman has lost 80 pounds, we pay little attention. "Yeah, well, she's white and all the diet plans and weight charts are geared toward her," we say, rolling our eyes. "What's that got to do with me?" If, however, the woman who has lost weight is a sista—even if her weight loss story is exactly the same as her white counterpart's—our ears perk up. "Hey, she's like me," we think. "I wonder how she did it." Dr. Kumanyika and I believe a database that tracks the weight loss success of African American women should be created. Although the National Institutes of Health has a large database of weight loss success stories, the percentage of black women is very small. The lack of a database that is specific to black women is too bad, because one look at the popularity of black women's weight loss stories in health magazines among other women of color tells us that such a database would go a long way toward improving our attitudes about losing weight.

Dr. Kumanyika also discovered that there are certain aspects of our lives that may make us more resistant to the idea of exercise than white women. For example, if we work at physically demanding jobs, we tend to want to collapse into our easy chairs at the end of the day and on weekends, too. Because many sistas do work at such jobs, whether as bus drivers, nurses, schoolteachers, waitresses, or salesclerks who are on their feet all day, and some of us even work two jobs, we can't imagine adding one more activity to our schedules. On the other hand, our white sisters, many of whom are in higher socioeconomic brackets, may be out riding bikes, working out at the gym, hiking, or canoeing to fill their weekend hours. One thing they have learned from experience is that keeping active replenishes your energy levels rather than draining them. Many times I've gone into the gym feeling exhausted and left an hour later feeling completely renewed.

Performing a Self-Assessment Test

Now that I've debunked the rationalizations that can derail your train to healthy living and (I hope) convinced you of the attitude adjustments you need to make in order to get your life on track, all you need to do is get started. A good first step is to perform a self-assessment test, not from a *looking*-good standpoint, but from a *feeling*-good one. If you answer yes to more than five of the questions below, know that you need to adopt my healthy living plan.

You Are as Well as You Feel

❖ Do you have frequent headaches or feel strange, unexplained pains in your chest, hips, abdomen, or back?
❖ Is your blood pressure elevated?
❖ Does climbing a flight of stairs leave you panting?
❖ Are you often too tired to engage in simple activities—bowling or clubbing with friends, going to concerts, catching a movie? Do you

spend most of your free time curled up in front of the TV?

✤ Do your joints ache?
✤ Do you often suffer from acid reflux (heartburn)?

You Are as Well as You Act

✤ Do you ignore advice to have your blood pressure and cholesterol levels checked?
✤ Do you smoke?
✤ Have you forgotten to have your blood sugar levels checked?
✤ Do you routinely have more than two drinks a day? (One drink equals 4 ounces of wine, 12 ounces of beer, or 1 and a half ounces of hard liquor.)

You Are as Fit as You Act

✤ Do you sit at your desk for eight hours without taking a lunchtime walk around the block or climbing the stairs during the course of your day?
✤ Are there many days when the only activity you do is the round-trip walk from the bedroom to the kitchen, the television, the bathroom, then back to bed?
✤ Do you usually walk less than a mile a day?
✤ Do you tend to avoid fun activities that require a good amount of energy, such as tennis, softball or baseball, dancing, martial

arts, swimming, biking, roller-skating, or ice skating?

✤ Do you spend fewer than two hours a week doing household chores such as laundry, vacuuming, mopping, or sweeping?

You Are What You Eat

✤ Do you routinely skip breakfast?

✤ When you do eat breakfast, is it usually bacon, eggs, toast or a muffin, and coffee?

✤ Do you eat when you're not hungry?

✤ Do you eat constantly while watching television?

✤ If you stop at a fast-food restaurant, does your meal look like a construction worker's lunch: cheesy double- or triple-decker sandwich, supersized fries, and a biggie drink?

✤ Do you think of a serving in terms of the giant-sized portions you're served in restaurants or fast-food places?

✤ Do you eat vegetables only three times a week, maybe one serving a day?

✤ Do lettuce, ketchup, and french fries count as vegetables in your meal plan?

✤ Do you drink half and half or cream in your coffee because it tastes better?

✤ Do you eat everything on your plate for the benefit of "Africa's starving children" or because you grew up in a house that wasted nothing?

❖ Are fruits and vegetables infrequent parts of your diet?

Studying your answers to these questions will help you change your focus from how you look in that cute outfit to your overall, long-term well-being. Once you make the connection between weight and your health, you'll be better prepared to make healthy lifestyle changes—for good.

Shaking Out Your Family Medical Tree

My self-assessment test is only the first step toward figuring out your healthy living picture. A family assessment could help, too, because while you may have your dad's big brown eyes, your mom's gorgeous legs, or Aunt Mamie's curvy hips, you could also have inherited a tendency toward a whole host of ailments from your family. Breast and colon cancer, heart disease, osteoporosis, and diabetes all have a genetic component to them, so it is wise to know your family medical history. A family medical history is a record of important medical information about your relatives. Knowing your family medical history can help you and your doctor determine potential health problems as well as allow you to take preventive measures to reduce your risk. You can begin your family history by talking with your immediate family—grandparents, parents, and siblings. Their health provides you with the most important information about genetic risks you may run.

If some of these relatives are deceased, it may take

some real detective work to find the desired information. Medical records, death certificates, newspaper obituaries, and old letters can be valuable sources of information for you to tap. I've also found that looking through old baby books, photo albums, or scrapbooks can provide visual clues to conditions such as obesity and osteoporosis. You might consider working on the medical history at the next family reunion, when many of your family members are all in the same place at one time. Every family has an unofficial historian who knows about the health and habits of previous generations. You might run into some resistance; you and I know that black people, especially members of the older generations, are often reluctant to discuss sensitive issues. If your family is like mine and many other African American families, medical secrets are tantamount to family secrets.

Take the example of Rosetta, my guardian, who lived with the painful secret of breast cancer for two years without telling anyone except her sister and without getting any treatment. She couldn't share such intimate information with anyone. I was a student at Virginia State University when I got a call from my uncle that I should come home that weekend, because Rosetta was in the hospital and in trouble. The ride to Hadley Memorial Hospital was completely silent; you really could hear a pin drop. All the while I was worried sick. I'd already lost one mother—how could this be happening to me again? Once we arrived at the hospital, Rosetta greeted me as she always did, with a broad smile. But I could see the pain radiating over her face. When we began to embrace, the nurse cautioned me, "Don't squeeze her." She had had a radical mastectomy. And because losing her breast was such a blow to her sense of womanhood, I'm sure that if my uncle hadn't called me, she would never have let me know.

Don't let the reluctance of your relatives to discuss their health problems prevent you from getting this information. Tell them how important it could be to your own health and that of future generations, too. Rosetta, of course, was not a blood relation of mine, so I tell this story only because I think her sense of secrecy is typical of the problems you may face trying to get a family medical history. But be persistent. Once you do get the facts, the picture they may paint could be all the encouragement you need to make potentially life-altering, health-enhancing changes in your lifestyle.

In my own case, there are factors of heredity that place me at a higher risk for hypertension, vascular problems (poor circulation), cancer, and weight problems, as you will see in the family medical tree I did tracing the illnesses and causes of death on my mother's side of the family (going back only as far as her parents). To create this tree, I used any sources of information I could get. For example, although I didn't know my mother's father, who died before I was born, I was able to recall stories that I had heard told over and over during many a family gathering, of my granddad, who suffered a massive stroke and as a result was barely able to carry on an audible conversation. And from personal observation I knew what had happened to two of my uncles, Linwood and Ben, strong, vibrant, independent men who took care of their families but who were later rendered almost helpless as a result of becoming amputees. For information about other aunts and uncles whom I hadn't known I had to rely on relatives, who were not always able to remember everything about the illnesses and causes of death among my mother's siblings. Still, I was able to create a complete enough family medical history to show me that I have good reason to maintain my weight at a normal level, get plenty of exercise, and pay particular attention to my diet. You may want to use the occasion of your next family reunion to start finding out your own reasons for making lifesaving changes.

Be as specific as you can when you gather this information. If possible, health histories should note the date of birth and the date and cause of death, as well as any serious medical diseases such as heart disease, stroke, diabetes, cancer, or glaucoma. Try to learn the age of onset of any diseases, because this can be a vital clue about your genetic predisposition. If, for example, your grandmother developed breast cancer at age 35, this information is much more of a warning sign than learning that she developed the disease at age 77. It may help if you draw a genealogical chart (see Dr. Ro's Medical Family Tree). This will let you track whether a disease has passed from generation to generation. If you notice the same diseases in different generations or a pattern developing, branch out and start obtaining information about cousins, aunts, and uncles; this will make your family medical history a more complete picture.

You can't change your genes, but you can present this information to your physician, and he or she can tailor your health plan or perform tests or screenings for diseases for which you are at risk earlier than he or she would have without this information.

Frequently Asked Questions

Q Dr. Ro: I want to start being more active, but there aren't enough hours in my day to fit in a 30-minute workout. How can I start some sort of exercise program?

A *Don't limit yourself to 30-minute exercise blocks if your day is too jam-packed for them. Instead, squeeze in three 10-minute sessions. Can't eke out 10 minutes? Take the stairs instead of the elevator at work. Use a few minutes of your lunch break to walk around the parking lot. At home, do a few push-ups, crunches, and jumping jacks. Find activities that have hidden exercise benefits, such as washing your car or doing laps around the mall when you go shopping. Just don't get caught in the trap of thinking that if you don't have time to do a full workout, you shouldn't do anything at all. Every little bit helps, even if all you do is park farther away from the store or do lunges as you vacuum the floor or push the baby in a stroller. Household chores such as sweeping and mopping and hobbies such as gardening are activities that burn calories, too.*

Dr. Ro's Medical Family Tree

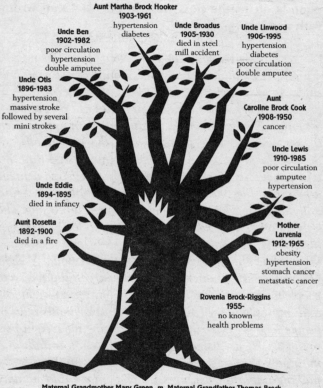

Aunt Martha Brock Hooker
1903-1961
hypertension
diabetes

Uncle Ben
1902-1982
poor circulation
hypertension
double amputee

Uncle Broadus
1905-1930
died in steel
mill accident

Uncle Linwood
1906-1995
hypertension
diabetes
poor circulation
double amputee

Uncle Otis
1896-1983
hypertension
massive stroke
followed by several
mini strokes

Aunt
Caroline Brock Cook
1908-1950
cancer

Uncle Lewis
1910-1985
poor circulation
amputee
hypertension

Uncle Eddie
1894-1895
died in infancy

Aunt Rosetta
1892-1900
died in a fire

Mother
Larvenia
1912-1965
obesity
hypertension
stomach cancer
metastatic cancer

Rovenia Brock-Riggins
1955-
no known
health problems

Maternal Grandmother Mary Green m. Maternal Grandfather Thomas Brock
1870-1963
glaucoma
followed by blindness

1859-1953
hypertension
massive stroke
followed by
mini strokes

Q   Dr. Ro: I hate exercising and I love my Big Macs and fries. My friends told me about a fabulous new diet that I could lose 30 pounds on in the next month. So what's so wrong with that?

A   First, you should know that losing 30 pounds in a single month is not safe. It is safest to lose weight gradually at the rate of 1 to 2 pounds a week. That would equal, at best, 8 pounds in a month. Further, it would be difficult to maintain such a diet over the long haul to keep the weight off (see Secret 5 for my take on fad diets). Having said that, if I told you it was possible to lose weight or even to achieve a healthful lifestyle without watching what you eat and without getting your booty on the move, I'd be lying. The only way to achieve long-term weight loss success is through a combination of eating less and exercising more—and the proof of that is in the National Weight Control Registry, which is one of the largest databases of people who have made a success of long-term weight loss and maintenance. The database tracks thousands of people who get it when it comes to losing the weight permanently. Eighty percent of people who drop pounds and maintain the weight loss over the long haul do so by making important changes in food intake and activity levels. As for that miracle weight loss diet, see Secret 3!

Q   Dr. Ro: I know I didn't develop my unhealthy lifestyle overnight, but I've been determined to solve the problem lickety-split. But all I've gotten from this quick-fix attitude is frustration. What will really help me reach my weight loss and health goals?

A   *By now you know there are no shortcuts to permanent weight loss and good health, so do yourself a favor and throw out all of the old garbage you have stored over the years that says anything to the contrary. Like any other goal in life, weight loss takes some sacrifice and commitment. It takes dedication and, pretty often, hard work. Sticking with your commitment will ensure years of long and productive life. But you must first commit to a new mind-set. Start by writing down your weight loss goals. Why do you want to lose weight? How much do you want to lose? Focus on your internal motivation for losing weight—getting healthy or feeling better—because this tends to lead to long-term success. External motivators such as getting into that slinky dress for the company's Christmas party, though powerful, tend to be short-lived.*

Q   Dr. Ro: How can I get my friends and family to help me stick to my goals?

A   *Tell family and close friends your intentions. Enlist their help. Sure, you could go it alone, but having a support system makes it easier to stay on track. Grab a buddy to help you stay motivated when* you exercise. These actions say you're serious about your commitment to a new lifestyle.

Q Dr. Ro: Every year I make living healthier one of my New Year's resolutions. By February 1, that resolution has been forgotten. How can I implement my plan and, more important, stick to it?

A Understand that moving from an unhealthy lifestyle to a healthy one is a multistage process. Here's a guide to doing it step by step: (1) Decide you want to make a change. In your case, this has become a yearly resolution, so you obviously do. (2) Assess your health status, using the guidelines I provided above so that you'll know if you need to eat more healthfully, become more active, or deal with any illnesses that may be threatening you. (3) Decide on your long-term goals: Do you want to lose weight? How much? Or maybe you just want to lose inches and gain strength. Or maybe you look fine now but want to change your bad eating habits before they catch up to you. (4) Whatever your goals are, write them in a journal and tell your friends and family your plans. (5) Enlist the aid of your husband, your kids, and your best sista-friend to stick to your guns, then include these people in your plan. After all, they need healthier lifestyles, too. (6) Start small—if you've been completely sedentary, don't expect to run five miles the first day you head to the track. Begin at whatever level you can, and build on that, increasing the duration and intensity of your exercise in the weeks to come. The main thing is to make a start, however modest. Remember, it takes only three weeks to develop a habit.

Secret

Your Sista-Body Really Is
Something Special: Get It Movin'!

In Secret 1 we talked about how we have to change our attitudes in order to lead healthier lives. In this secret I'll tell you how our sista-bodies are different from white women's bodies—in both good and bad ways—and how those differences can mean the difference between living long, productive, healthy lives and dying early. We'll learn how to measure our fitness status and what the risk factors are for certain diseases—risk factors that can be exacerbated by excess weight. We'll also learn how to use exercise to reduce those risk factors.

Good News

For starters, you should know that though women of all races are in most ways genetically similar, there *are* some differences between our bodies and those of white women. According to the Body Composition

Laboratory at Baylor College of Medicine, black women have greater bone mass, and greater bone mass means stronger bones. Premenopausal black women have, on average, about 10 to 12 percent more bone mass and also more muscle mass, for the more bone you have, the more muscle you have. This is a terrific advantage, not only because it makes you stronger, but because the greater your muscle mass, the faster and more efficiently your body burns calories (larger muscles need more fuel, and calories are the fuel).

The calorie-burning effect of muscle is further intensified by exercise. Unfortunately, black women tend not to exercise. So our bone and muscle advantage is offset by our inactivity (and also by our diets), with the result that we end up carrying more body fat than our white counterparts. And all those extra muscles you have will soon atrophy if you don't work them. Need proof? Think about those sagging pouches of flesh on the backs of your arms, which seemed to develop overnight. These flapping "wings" are the direct result of not working the triceps muscles.

Bad News

There is an interesting body of research by a group of German scientists at the University of Essen, who have identified a gene called the thrifty gene, which they believe enables people to withstand starvation. Dr. Francine Kaufman, a prominent endocrinologist at Children's Hospital in Los Angeles, agrees that this gene may have been the reason so many African slaves were able to survive the Middle Passage. The thrifty gene helps the body make as much use as possible of a minimal amount of food. Unfortunately, today's descendants of those slaves still have that gene, even though starvation is no longer a threat. The typical sedentary lifestyle and high-fat, high-calorie diet of many African Americans jump-starts this gene, with the result that obesity and its attendant diseases—including coronary artery disease, hypertension, and diabetes—have become a major health problem. Put simply, our bodies, designed to withstand starvation, can't handle the increased calories and fat that are the hallmarks of a life of plenty.

Researchers studying this thrifty gene have found that overweight people are three times as likely as their slimmer cousins to carry two copies of this gene (one from each parent). And women who carry two copies are six times more likely to retain excess weight after pregnancy than those who have one copy of the gene or none at all.

Here's something else to think about: Researchers have found that because of a slower energy metabolism, obese black sistas burn fewer calories a day at rest than their white sisters. Sounds like a raw deal? Maybe, but knowing this will at least allow you to do something about it, and I'll have plenty of suggestions to help you in this chapter and every other chapter in the book.

There's more in the bad news department—having to do not with genes but with cultural and socioeconomic factors. We're socialized in our culture to turn to food for everything. A family member got a promotion? We celebrate with food. Someone dies? The table is laden with all manner of eats. Weddings, graduations, anniversaries—you name it, anytime we get together somebody will make sure we "get our eat on." Couple that with the fact that we're not usually preparing all that celebratory food in a healthy manner, and you've got a recipe for obesity. Add to that the low self-esteem and feelings of impotence, tension, anger, and stress that come from living in a racist society, and we're visiting the refrigerator even when we're not hungry.

Still need more proof that your sista-body is different? Did you know that we are less likely than women of all other races (except Hispanic women) to exercise? Heck, according to some researchers, we even think of working out as an added stress factor in our lives! And for the record, we (and many of our men) like our butts, hips, and thighs just the way they are, thank you very much. In one study of 500 black women in Washington, D.C., researchers at the Penn State College of Medicine and Center for Biostatistics and Epidemiology found that husbands and boyfriends of more than half of the women studied said they liked the weight their women carried on their bodies.

Weight Gain in the Sistahood

Check this out: 50 percent of black women (versus only about 25 percent of our white counterparts) are overweight between the ages of 20 and 44. According to the Centers for Disease Control and Prevention (CDC), as of the years 1999 and 2000, over one in two black women age 40 and over is obese. And black women are particularly likely to gain weight between the ages of 25 and 34—largely because of childbirth. Our weight gain during these key childbearing years is much higher than for white women. Why? Because we sistas tend to be of lower socioeconomic and educational status, and women in that situation tend to have more children and to eat a worse diet and to exercise less. And given the weight-retaining action of the thrifty gene, after the births of those children the weight is harder for us to lose than for white women. One reason this is particularly alarming is that women who gain significant amounts of weight around age 30 are believed to be at increased risk of breast cancer and probably other diseases as well. And if much of that fat is concentrated in the belly region, there is particular cause for concern. You'll discover as you read on (see pages 55, 63, and 70) the specific details of the health risks associated with abdominal weight gain.

Finding Our Way: Preventable Diseases

Although I like to think I'm providing my readers with secrets to a healthier life, it's no secret that black people are dying needlessly from diseases that are partly or largely related to the way we live—in other words, diseases that are at least partly preventable. But we're not doing a good job of prevention. We have a long history of not just eating too much sweet, high-fat, salty food, but of smoking too many cigarettes, sitting when we should be moving, and avoiding regular doctor visits. And that's just part of our problem.

Many of us shoulder economic burdens people of other races can only imagine, along with the tremendous stress of living in a racist society. It's no surprise, then, that we have a 38 percent higher chance of suffering a fatal heart attack than white women. In fact, more of us die from heart disease than from any other disease. Nearly one-third of all black women suffer from high blood pressure, and one in five of our deaths is due to hypertension. One in four of us age 55 and older has diabetes, and we're more likely than our white counterparts to develop complications related to diabetes, including kidney failure, blindness, heart disease, and even amputations. We are nearly three times as likely to die from a stroke, twice as likely to die from breast or cervical cancer. Is it any wonder our bodies need an extra dose of tender loving care? So please, as you read through these and the other grim statistics I'll be presenting in the next few pages, keep in mind that if you *do* give your body the care it deserves, these problems can to a large extent be prevented—and often reversed. It's up to you to do something about them.

Heart Disease

The Bad News ✦ Heart disease, also known as coronary heart disease or CHD, is the number one cause of death for women, killing roughly 500,000 each year. Half of those deaths are the direct result of heart attacks; the rest are related to the many complications suffered by those with heart disease. And, sistas, we are 69 percent more likely than our white counterparts to suffer heart disease and heart attacks, with an almost

70 percent greater risk of dying of heart disease. The American Heart Association reports that in the year 2000, the death rate from CHD among black women was 187 per 100,000 deaths compared to 145 per 100,000 deaths for white women. We are also more likely to get heart disease at an earlier age, and also to die of a heart attack at an earlier age than white women (some of us as young as 30)—facts that have only recently become known.

Actually, most all of the facts cited above about women and heart disease are relatively new to our awareness. So I guess you could say that they *were* secrets, although nobody meant to keep them secret—it's just that nobody had done the research to bring them to light.

The thinking for years, according to the experts, was that estrogen provided such good protection from heart disease in women until they reached menopause that they didn't need to worry about heart disease. Physicians were even taught that women, specifically black women, rarely had heart attacks. Though this way of thinking is changing—most doctors, for instance, are now much more aware that heart disease does occur in women—getting the message across to women themselves is taking a while.

The Good News ✦ According to the Centers for Disease Control, the incidence of heart disease and stroke can be drastically reduced by minimizing the risk factors for them—such as high blood pressure, high blood cholesterol, tobacco use, diabetes, physical inactivity, and a poor diet. For example, a 12 percent reduction in LDL cholesterol (the "bad" cholesterol) and a 25 percent increase in HDL cholesterol (the "good" cholesterol), which can usually be achieved via a healthful diet and daily exercise, can cut your heart disease and stroke risk in half.

Hypertension

The Bad News ✦ Hypertension, commonly called high blood pressure, is a condition in which the pressure of the blood as it is pumped through your arteries becomes abnormally high. Hypertension is a problem because it is a risk factor for so many other serious conditions, including heart disease, kidney failure, stroke, heart attack, and kidney damage, and because it is symptomless—many people don't know they have it. If we could just get our blood pressure under control, it would make a huge difference in the health of black folks—women in particular—because it afflicts our people in disproportionately high numbers. Nearly 37 percent of black women 20 and older have high blood pressure compared to 20 percent of white women. It is well known that black people suffer disproportionately from hypertension and stroke compared to whites. But you might wonder why this is so.

One reason is that high blood pressure is twice as common in obese women. Remember that black women have disproportionately high rates of obesity. Some scientists believe another part of the answer may be found in a genetic link. It seems the culprit could again be that thrifty gene, which may have helped African slaves to survive the Middle Passage not just through its weight-retaining properties but because it had sodium-retaining properties as well. The theory is that when those Africans were being transported to this country on the slave ships, forced to suffer inhumane living conditions, deprived of adequate food and water, and afflicted with diarrhea and seasickness that depleted their nutrients, those endowed with the sodium-retaining properties of the thrifty gene were better able to survive. Dr. Clarence Grim of the Charles Drew/UCLA Hypertension Center in Los Angeles believes that because those slaves whose bodies could hold on to salt were more likely to survive, they passed that genetic trait on to future generations. However, the same genetic trait that protected us hundreds of years ago has the opposite effect in the face of today's diet of highly processed, high-sodium foods, because our bodies need only a small amount of sodium to function under normal conditions. In people who are salt-sensitive, as many African Americans are, excess sodium causes fluid retention, which increases the volume of blood flowing through their veins and therefore increases blood pressure.

Another problem leading to hypertension is that we eat too many foods full of saturated fat and cholesterol. The fatty deposits left by these foods clog the arteries and cause atherosclerosis, which is also a factor in hypertension.

Finally, after many studies documenting the links between stress and hypertension, it is now acknowledged that high stress levels are a major factor, too. This is of particular interest to African Americans, who live in what is still a racist society and suffer unusually high levels of stress, which are now believed to play a significant role in the disproportionate rate at which African Americans suffer from hypertension.

The Good News: ✦ As I'm sure you've noticed by now, the good news about all the conditions I've been describing is right there in the bad news—because there's always something we can do about it. Since we African Americans are particularly vulnerable to the effects of salt on high blood pressure, for example, we can bypass the salt shaker and try to limit our salt intake to the recommended 2,400 mg of sodium per day, which is about 1⅓ teaspoons—or, better yet, to the 1,500 mg of sodium (⅔ teaspoon) that the low-salt Dietary Approaches to Stop Hypertension (DASH) eating plan has shown to be even more effective at lowering blood pressure. The low-salt DASH diet is also low in saturated fat, cholesterol, and total fat, while being high in fruits, vegetables, low-fat dairy foods, whole grains, and beans.

By losing 20 pounds, you can shave an average of 10 points off your systolic blood pressure (which is the first number that appears in your blood pressure reading) and 8 points from your diastolic pressure (the second number). What's more, getting a move on works, too. According to the CDC, a sedentary lifestyle accounts for 12 percent of hypertension cases in the United States. But that doesn't have to be your fate. Even people with moderately high blood pressure can lower it by 10 points (systolic and diastolic) by just walking a minimum of 20 minutes five days a week.

Finally, while there's little to be done in the immediate run about racism, we can try to take control of our response to it and thereby lower our stress levels. We can begin by making the active decision to take better care of ourselves. The combination of eating better and taking long walks or working out is a source of empowerment that rests on us.

Diabetes

Diabetes (sometimes called "sugar" in the black community) develops when the pancreas does not make enough insulin or the body does not use insulin correctly. Since insulin is the hormone that controls blood sugar levels and helps sugar enter the cells, where it is converted to energy, it is absolutely critical to our health and well-being. There are two types of diabetes. Type I is often referred to as "juvenile diabetes," although you do not have to be a child to develop it. A person who has this form makes little or no insulin and must have insulin injections. Type II, the more common type, is sometimes called "adult-onset diabetes," although both children and adults can get it. People with this type make insulin but either they do not make enough of it or their bodies have become resistant to its effects—a condition called insulin resistance.

Type II diabetes usually does not require insulin injections in the early stages; it can be controlled (or better yet, prevented) by diet and lifestyle changes.

The Bad News: ✦ The rate of diabetes has tripled in the African American community in the past 30 years. Nearly 12 percent of African American women 20 years of age and older have type II diabetes; 25 percent over age 55 have it. Approximately 2.8 million, or 13 percent, of all African Americans have diabetes, yet one-third of them do not know it.

The Good News: ✦ Improving your diet and lifestyle by becoming more physically active can make the difference between becoming diabetic and not. Did you know that if you are overweight and achieve a 5 to 7 percent weight loss, you can prevent or delay the onset of type II diabetes, even if you are at high risk for the disease? Just as in the case of heart disease, hypertension, and stroke, we now know that there is a lot we can do to prevent type II diabetes. Even though there is a genetic component, it is perhaps more preventable than previously thought. It is possible to reduce your risk of type II diabetes by incorporating lifestyle changes such as walking for 30 minutes a day, 5 days a week and, if needed, losing 10 to 15 pounds. Although the jury is still out as to how much you can reduce your risk, there's no question that taking a proactive stance toward such lifestyle issues as nutrition and exercise will benefit you.

Breast Cancer

Many African American women have heard that breast cancer is more common in their community. But nationwide studies suggest that, overall, the life-long chances of having breast cancer are similar for African American women and white women, with white women having a slightly higher incidence of developing the disease. African American women are slightly more likely than white women to develop breast cancer before age 50 and slightly less likely to develop breast cancer after age 50.

The Bad News: ✦ According to the National Cancer Institute, even though white women have a slightly higher incidence of breast cancer, African American women are more likely to die of it. In fact, they have the highest breast cancer death rates of *any* group. Many studies have been carried out in an attempt to understand why this is so. Some have even wondered if breast cancer in African American women is somehow fundamentally different from breast cancer in other groups. Though no basic differences have been found, one well-known fact is that African American women tend to be diagnosed with breast cancer at later stages, when the tumors are larger and have spread beyond the breast to the lymph nodes and other parts of the body. When breast cancers are found at more advanced stages, they are more difficult to treat, and survival rates are lower. There is also more evidence for the increased risk of developing breast cancer if the woman has gained significant weight in her midsection, becoming what we call "apple-shaped." Her risk is increased by two and a half times—*and* she is two and a half times more likely to die of the disease—if she gains belly fat around age 30, according to a study published in an issue of the journal *Cancer.* Another study, published in the *American Journal of Epidemiology*, showed that apple-shaped women were 34 percent more likely to develop breast cancer than thin pear-shaped women.

The Good News: ✦ Again, the consistent message appears to be that controlling lifestyle factors such as diet, exercise, and weight—and, of course, not smoking and not abusing alcohol or drugs—means you are much more likely to have a long and healthy life. Remember: Though some of the causes of the chronic illnesses and high mortality rates that plague our community remain obscure, it is clear that obesity and a sedentary lifestyle both play a part. And while there are plenty of things you can't change—not just racism but your family history and crime—lifestyle factors are within your power.

Fit Versus Fat

Don't think I'm only pointing the finger at my fat sistas; the truth is, you can be a size 4, unfit, and out of shape, or a size 16 or larger and quite fit.

Becky's Story: ✦ At 5 feet 7 inches and 182 pounds, fitness coach Becky Johnson could definitely be considered overweight. Always a curvy individual—"I started developing breasts in third grade," she says—Becky never dropped all of the weight she gained while she was pregnant with her daughter. A bad divorce and the struggle to keep a roof over her and her teenage daughter's heads helped add an additional 50 pounds, until she found herself tipping the scales at nearly 270 pounds. "I knew I had to get my weight under control," she says. "High blood pressure runs in my family, and I didn't want to have a stroke the way my mother and several of my aunts had."

Table 2-1. Obesity-Related Diseases and Their Complications

Obesity-Related Disease	Black Women Statistics	Complications
Hypertension	*One-third of all black women have high blood pressure*	*Increased risk of heart disease and stroke*
Heart disease	*Black women are 69 percent more likely than white women to suffer heart disease and heart attacks*	*70 percent more likely to die from heart disease; increased risk of stroke*
Breast cancer	*Black women are less likely than white women to discover they have the disease, more likely than white women to be diagnosed at a later stage, and more likely to die of it than women of any other racial or ethnic group*	*One in three black women diagnosed with breast cancer dies*

Obesity-Related Disease	Black Women Statistics	Complications
Diabetes	*Fourth leading cause of death among black women; four to six times more common in blacks than in whites; one in four black women 50 and older has diabetes, but half of them don't know it; 32 percent of black women ages 65–74 have diabetes*	*Increased risk of kidney failure, blindness, amputations, heart disease, stroke*
Cervical cancer	*Fifth most common cancer in African American women*	*Infertility, hysterectomy; twice the risk of dying from the disease as white women*
Stroke	*Blacks are two times more likely than whites to suffer strokes*	*Paralysis and death; three times the risk of dying from stroke as white women*

Becky had changed her eating habits years before; her ex-husband was a vegetarian, and she stopped eating pork and fried foods during their marriage. Still, working two jobs left little time for exercise, and at 32 she found that diet alone didn't help her drop many pounds. But then something changed. "I signed up for a spinning class, and fell in love," she says. It was in that spinning class, scheduled in the early mornings before heading off to her full-time gig, that Becky discovered a new passion: fitness. "I added a kickboxing class on weekends, and I started to see a change almost immediately. It was like the pounds were melting off. My daughter, my co-workers, everybody I knew kept telling me how good I looked. That made me want to work out even more."

But her schedule was already full. So two years into her new lifestyle, Becky made the drastic decision to quit her part-time job and work toward a personal trainer certification. It meant a bit of belt tightening for a while, but Becky stuck with it because exercising gave her a high and she wanted to share that with other women. "Before I got finished with my certification and got my first client, I added jogging to my own fitness regimen." By this time Becky had dropped to 182 pounds. And there she plateaued.

"At first I was angry. I was working out like crazy, but the weight loss just stopped," Becky says. "Then I realized that I am in fabulous cardiovascular shape. I can run 10 miles. Though other people may think I'm fat, I'm actually very fit." And she is. Six years after starting her quest, Becky is a fitness coach who teaches spinning, aerobics, kickboxing, and boot-camp classes at a gym, and she has a full stable of personal-training clients. In addition to the personal training and teaching classes, Becky squeezes in six-mile runs three times a week. She still hasn't budged from 182 pounds.

But at 182 pounds, Becky can run faster and jump higher than many of her peers, and she has amazing energy and endurance, too, because of her remarkable fitness. In other words, you don't have to shorten your life span just because you don't look like a model.

Assessing Your Risk Factors

Being fit means more than just having great cardio output. It is also associated with having normal blood pressure, good cholesterol, and healthy blood sugar levels, all of which Becky has. It also involves understanding and knowing your aerobic training zone, basal metabolic rate, and body mass index, all of which will be explained below.

Blood Pressure

Blood pressure is a measurement of the force applied against the walls of the arteries as the heart pumps blood through the body. The pressure is determined by the force and amount of blood pumped and the size and flexibility of the arteries. A reading consists of two numbers, for example, 110/70, which is said as "110 over 70." According to the Joint National Committee on Prevention, Detection, Evaluation and Treatment of High Blood Pressure (JNC), a normal blood pressure level is now 115/75 for an adult. After that you are considered pre-hypertensive with a BP of 120/80. Of course, your blood pressure is measured as part of any routine physical exam. You can also buy a kit for as little as $20 and measure your blood pressure at home. If you are checking your own pressure, make sure to measure it while in a seated position with your arm at the same level as your heart, after you have been at rest for five minutes or more, when you are relaxed.

Cholesterol

Cholesterol is a waxy, fatlike substance that occurs naturally in your body. Your body needs it to function normally. In the right amounts and the right kind—the "good" cholesterol—it's a good thing.

What we mean when we say "good" cholesterol is HDL (high-density lipoprotein), which removes cholesterol from your bloodstream and carries it back to the liver, where it passes from the body. "Bad" cholesterol or LDL (low-density lipoprotein), on the other hand, brings cholesterol *to* the cells. When too much LDL cholesterol circulates in the blood, it can slowly build up in the walls of the arteries that feed your heart, clogging them. This condition is known as atherosclerosis. If a clot forms where the plaque is, the blood flow to part of the heart can be blocked, causing a heart attack. If a clot blocks blood flow to part of the brain, a stroke results. Some experts think that HDL cholesterol can counteract this potential danger by removing cholesterol from atherosclerotic plaque, thus slowing the buildup.

Women tend to have cholesterol levels that stay below 200 milligrams per deciliter (mg/dl) until they approach menopause, when falling estrogen levels often cause cholesterol to rise to an unhealthy 220–240 mg/dl or higher.

Be forewarned—knowing your total cholesterol is one thing, but it is also important to know your LDL,

HDL, and triglyceride levels in order to more accurately understand your risk for heart disease. According to the National Heart, Lung, and Blood Institute, desirable levels for your lipids are:

Total cholesterol:	Less than 200 mg/dl
LDL:	Less than 100 mg/dl
HDL:	More than 40 mg/dl
Triglycerides:	Less than 150 mg/dl

But keep in mind that even more important than total cholesterol is the ratio of total cholesterol to HDL, because high levels of HDL are protective against heart disease. Any ratio under 4.5 is good—the lower the better. Imagine a woman with a high total cholesterol of 240, but also a high HDL of 80. Her ratio of total cholesterol to HDL is 3 (240 divided by 80), indicating a lower risk, not the higher risk you might imagine given the total cholesterol reading.

The National Heart, Lung, and Blood Institute recommends that all women 20 and older have their cholesterol checked through a small blood sample every five years. A complete lipid profile, which consists of measurements of your blood levels of LDL (or bad) cholesterol, HDL (or good) cholesterol, and triglycerides (stored fat), will determine if your levels fall within a normal range. The lipid profile is measured by a fasting lipoprotein test, taken when you have not eaten for a prescribed amount of time—usually between 9 and 12 hours.

Blood Sugar

Usually blood sugar is measured by testing a drop of blood collected during a finger-prick test. A healthy blood sugar level should range from 70 mg/dl to 120 mg/dl. A level higher than 140 mg/dl may indicate diabetes.

But diabetes isn't the only thing that blood sugar measurements tell us about. You may also have heard about syndrome X. The term was first used by a group of Stanford University scientists to describe a cluster of conditions, including high blood pressure, elevated blood sugar, high triglycerides, low HDL, and excess abdominal fat (the so-called apple shape), which tend to appear together in some people and increase their risk for diabetes, heart disease, stroke, and fatty deposits in the liver. Syndrome X sometimes goes by other names. Researchers at the Centers for Disease Control and Prevention refer to this condition as metabolic syndrome. African American people and Hispanic people appear more likely to have metabolic syndrome than people of other races, and African American women were more likely to have it (26 percent) than African American men (16 percent). But since the syndrome is caused by improper nutrition and lack of exercise, diet and exercise can help to return the metabolism to normal.

Syndrome X is closely linked to insulin resistance. In fact, insulin resistance is one of its defining factors. Again, insulin is the hormone responsible for getting energy, in the form of glucose (blood sugar), into our cells. An insulin-resistant person has cells that, for reasons not fully understood, don't respond effectively to the action of insulin. The result is that after eating, a person with insulin resistance will have elevated levels of glucose circulating in the blood, signaling yet more insulin to be released from the pancreas until the glucose is taken up by the cells. Experts believe about 10 to 25 percent of the adult population may be resistant to insulin.

Aerobic Capacity

Fitness refers to your cardiovascular or aerobic capacity—that is, your heart, lung, and circulatory system's ability to supply oxygen-rich blood to your muscles and organs. Your aerobic capacity is based on how efficiently your body can deliver oxygen to your muscles and how much oxygen your muscles can use for energy. In other words, it is a measure of the maximum rate at which oxygen can be taken up and utilized by the body during exercise. Typically a person's aerobic capacity is measured by having her walk briskly or jog on a treadmill, at a gradually increasing rate of intensity, up to the point at which oxygen consumption plateaus and shows no further increase with additional workload (also called maximum oxygen consumption, expressed as the formula VO_{2max}). This is a test usually ordered by a doctor if there is a suspicion of heart ailment, and it is done with special equipment in a medical lab or the doctor's office.

Regular exercising at a specific level and for a certain time will help improve your aerobic capacity. The key is to exercise at an intensity that is within your aerobic training zone for a minimum of 20 minutes three times a week. Though most of us won't have occasion to undergo the specialized testing that measures aerobic capacity, all of us can measure our aerobic training zone. To figure your aerobic training zone, subtract your age from 220. The resulting figure is your maximum heart rate. Multiply this number by 65 percent for the lower end of the training range and by 85 percent for the upper end of the range.

Here's my own example. At age 46, my maximum heart rate is

$$220 - 46 = 174$$
$$174 \times .65 = 113.1$$
$$174 \times .85 = 147.9$$

Therefore, if I aim to remain in my aerobic training zone, my heart rate should be between 113 and 148 beats per minute when I'm doing an aerobic exercise that challenges it. You can count those beats by putting a finger to your pulse. Or you may be able to use a monitor. The exercise machines in many gyms can monitor your heart rate. You can also buy your own pulse monitor, often in the form of a wristwatch and chest band, but these pulse monitors can be expensive.

BMI and Obesity

So how should we measure ourselves? Most experts agree that body mass index (BMI) is perhaps the best and easiest way to discover whether or not you're too heavy. There are more accurate measures of body fat— total body water, for example, or total body potassium—but they're expensive and not readily available.

BMI is a favored measure because it is simple to calculate, costs nothing, and is generally reliable.

Basically, the BMI is a weight assessment tool that evaluates your weight in relation to your height. Your BMI is a better measure of overweight and obesity than body weight alone, and it is a good predictor of your risk for disease. BMI is determined by dividing your weight in pounds by the square of your height in inches and multiplying by 703. Or—much easier— consult a BMI table such as the one I provide on page 68, where the calculations have all been done for you. All you need to do is plug in your weight and height.

The athletes among you, like Becky, should remember that while BMI is generally a good indicator of whether or not a woman is overweight, it does not take into consideration the ratio of muscle to fat. Because muscle weighs more than fat, it is possible for a healthy, well-muscled individual with very low body fat to be considered overweight using the BMI formula. But very few of us need to take this exception into account, since very few of us have a high ratio of muscle to fat.

So what does BMI have to do with health, you ask? A lot. Even though the experts can't seem to make up their minds about the exact numbers that indicate a weight problem, as I'll explain below, the bottom line is this: Once certain levels are reached, the higher your BMI, the greater your risk of certain conditions, such as coronary heart disease, type II diabetes, and high blood pressure.

Sizing Yourself with the BMI

Find out where you stand by consulting the body mass index (BMI) table below. Find your weight in the left-hand column, move across until you find your height, and then look at the figure where they intersect to arrive at your BMI. According to the most convincing knowledge to date, if you have a BMI of 25 or greater, you could be running a higher risk of getting the diseases that have been killing black people (especially black women). But now some experts are suggesting that BMIs should be considerably lower than 25. A study released in July 2001 found that people with BMIs between 22 and 24.9 were significantly more likely to develop gallstones, colon cancer, high blood pressure, and diabetes than adults with lower BMIs. So the authors of the study recommended that after age 18, we should maintain a BMI between 18.5 and 21.9.

But if a BMI that low seems impossible to you, then shoot for the higher number of 25. And remember what I've said about weight by itself. It could be possible that you don't need to lose pounds. You be the judge: If you can walk up and down stairs and go about your day without feeling exhausted, your blood sugar, blood pressure, and blood cholesterol levels are within the healthy range, and you're happy with the way you look, you must be doing something right, so give yourself credit for that.

Now, if you have a BMI of less than 18.5, you could be underweight. This means you'll have to increase your calories to maintain a healthier picture overall.

Table 2-2 Body Mass Index (BMI) Table

Height (Feet and Inches)

Weight (Pounds)	5'0"	5'1"	5'2"	5'3"	5'4"	5'5"	5'6"	5'7"	5'8"	5'9"	5'10"	5'11"	6'0"	6'1"	6'2"	6'3"	6'4"
100	20	19	18	18	17	17	16	16	15	15	14	14	14	13	13	12	12
105	21	20	19	19	18	17	17	16	16	16	15	15	14	14	13	13	13
110	21	21	20	19	19	18	18	17	17	16	16	15	15	15	14	14	13
115	22	22	21	20	20	19	19	18	17	17	17	16	16	15	15	14	14
120	23	23	22	21	21	20	19	19	18	18	17	17	16	16	15	15	15
125	24	24	23	22	21	21	20	20	19	18	18	17	17	16	16	16	15
130	25	25	24	23	22	22	21	20	20	19	19	18	18	17	17	16	16
135	26	26	25	24	23	22	22	21	21	20	19	19	18	18	17	17	16
140	27	26	26	25	24	23	23	22	21	21	20	20	19	18	18	17	17
145	28	27	27	26	25	24	23	23	22	21	21	20	20	19	19	18	18
150	29	28	27	27	26	25	24	23	23	22	22	21	20	20	19	19	18
155	30	29	28	27	27	26	25	24	24	23	22	22	21	20	20	19	19
160	31	30	29	28	27	27	26	25	24	24	23	22	22	21	21	20	19
165	32	31	30	29	28	27	27	26	25	24	24	23	22	22	21	21	20
170	33	32	31	30	29	28	27	27	26	25	24	24	23	22	22	21	21
175	34	33	32	31	30	29	28	27	27	26	25	24	24	23	22	22	21
180	35	34	33	32	31	30	29	28	27	27	26	25	24	24	23	22	22
185	36	35	34	33	32	31	30	29	28	27	27	26	25	24	24	23	23
190	37	36	35	34	33	32	31	30	29	28	27	26	26	25	24	24	23
195	38	37	36	35	33	32	31	31	30	29	28	27	26	26	25	24	24
200	39	38	37	35	34	33	32	31	30	30	29	28	27	26	26	25	24
205	40	39	37	36	35	34	33	32	31	30	29	29	28	27	26	26	25
210	41	40	38	37	36	35	34	33	32	31	30	29	28	28	27	26	26
215	42	41	39	38	37	36	35	34	33	32	31	30	29	28	28	27	26
220	43	42	40	39	38	37	36	34	33	32	32	31	30	29	28	27	27
225	44	43	41	40	39	37	36	35	34	33	32	31	31	30	29	28	27
230	45	43	42	41	39	38	37	36	35	34	33	32	31	30	30	29	28
235	46	44	43	42	40	39	38	37	36	35	34	33	32	31	30	29	29
240	47	45	44	43	41	40	39	38	36	35	34	33	33	32	31	30	29
245	48	46	45	43	42	41	40	38	37	36	35	34	33	32	31	31	30
250	49	47	46	44	43	42	40	39	38	37	36	35	34	33	32	31	30

☐ Underweight ▨ Weight Appropriate ☐ Overweight ▨ Obese

We'll talk about the particulars of that in chapters to come.

Remember: The CDC recommends that you check your BMI every two years to make sure you're staying on track. Just know that BMI is a tool and don't get freaked out if yours is too high or low. You can make subtle changes to improve your condition, and that, my sista, is exactly why I'm here.

Pears Versus Apples: The Shape of Diseases to Come

BMI aside, recent studies indicate that body fat is still a good predictor of what a person's health risk may be. Women are particularly cautioned to keep body fat percentages low. Some researchers maintain that women who are apple-shaped rather than pear-shaped—that is, who carry most of their fat in their upper body (around their waist or in their abdomen) rather than below it and who have a waist measurement of more than 35 inches—are at increased risk for developing breast cancer, as are women who gain significant amounts of abdominal weight around age 30. A study from the H. Lee Moffitt Cancer Center and Research Institute at the University of South Florida in Tampa found that these same women also have a higher incidence of dying from breast cancer once they get it. The apple-shaped body with its extra weight around the midsection has also been linked to a greater risk of developing heart disease, diabetes, high blood pressure, gallbladder disease, and stroke—independent even of BMI.

There's more. A group of researchers at Yale

University looked at 59 premenopausal women and concluded that the way your body responds to stress may be related to the tendency to continue to gain weight in the belly region. The apple-shaped women in the study secreted more of a hormone called cortisol when they were subjected to highly stressful situations than the pear-shaped women. This finding is interesting because cortisol may activate an enzyme that makes fat cells larger. Translation? You get fatter in the belly region. The Yale researchers concluded that getting plenty of exercise and sleep in order to lower stress might be good ammunition in the battle of the bulge. The message we get from all of these data, conflicting as they may sometimes appear to be, is to keep your weight under control. Since weight gain in adulthood is often a factor in abdominal fat, women should try very hard to keep those added pounds from creeping up on them. (See how in Secret 5, page 151).

Metabolism 101

Before we move from the couch into an action-packed lifestyle, let's have a sit-down about your metabolism. It's important to understand it in order to be able to lose weight if necessary. I'd also like to dispel a couple of metabolism-related myths that sistas seem to believe. Let's begin with the basics.

Simply put, metabolism is the process by which the food you eat is converted into the energy you need. Whether slow or fast, your metabolism is the necessary engine that keeps the car (your body) running and it can be expressed in number form. The basal metabolic rate (BMR) is the amount of calories you burn at rest—in other words, it's the number of calories you burn just to keep breathing and to keep your heart beating. A number of factors affect actual BMRs for specific individuals. For example, a lean person with a relatively high muscle-to-fat ratio burns more calories at rest than a person who carries more fat on her body.

Here are a few other BMR facts for you to consider:

❧ Your BMR decreases when you go on a diet that has fewer calories than your normal diet. In response to fewer calories, the body lowers its BMR because it thinks there is a famine. This is why you often experience the "plateau effect" when dieting—losing a certain amount of weight when you first go on a diet, but then not being able to lose any more.

❧ Your BMR increases in response to increased physical activity. Not only do we use up calories during exercise, but the increased BMR continues even after we have finished exercising, often for several hours. The amount of increase varies from person to person, but even a modest increase should counteract the body's tendency to decrease BMR when we cut calories. We don't know the exact reason physical exercise leads to an increased BMR. Experts theorize that the higher metabolic rate may be due to the possibility that exercise burns fat while preserving more of our lean body tissue, and higher proportions of lean body tissue burn calories more effectively.

❧ Exercise is the only effective way to increase your BMR. Many diets claim to increase metabolic rate through special fat-burning foods, but don't believe the hype—the truth is, there are no such foods. Your metabolic rate falls if you start dieting and start to shed excess pounds, and while you may be able to counteract that fall by increased exercise, there is no evidence whatsoever that eating any particular food can make your metabolic rate higher than it was before you dieted.

❖ A low BMR does not cause obesity. Except in the rare cases of serious metabolic illness, it is not possible to blame your metabolism for obesity. Your metabolism certainly has an effect on how much you weigh, but the main reasons for obesity lie elsewhere.

Calculating Your Daily Caloric Requirements

To estimate the total number of calories your body needs per day, there's a formula you can use to calculate your approximate BMR and determine the calories needed just to sustain basic life processes.

Using this simple formula, I will plug in my own weight, height, and age numbers, to show you how it is done.

Formula:
655 + (4.4 × weight in pounds) + (4.7 × height in inches) − (4.7 × age)

Formula with my figures:
655 + (4.4 × **126 pounds**) + (4.7 × **63 inches**) − (4.7 × **46 years**)

655 + (554.4) + (296.1) − (216.2) = 1,289 calories per day, minimum

Next, in order to determine *actual* daily caloric needs, I must factor in my activity level by multiplying my basic calorie requirement of 1,289 by a figure from one of the categories below:

0.9 if you are inactive and have crash-dieted frequently during the past two years

1.2 if you are inactive

1.3 if you are moderately active (exercise three days per week or equivalent)

1.7 if you are very active

1.9 if you are extremely active

As a moderately active person, I multiply 1,289 × 1.3 = 1,676, or approximately 1,700 calories per day. If I were very active or extremely active, I would require more calories. On the other hand, if I were sedentary, I would require fewer calories per day. This formula approximates energy needs for normal daily body function, not for weight loss. If you are trying to lose weight, subtract 300–500 calories per day from your total energy needs, being truthful and realistic about your activity level.

Bringing the Numbers Together

Being fit means having all of these numbers fall within accepted limits. Meet that criteria, even if you are heavy, and you significantly reduce your risk for high blood pressure, stroke, heart disease, and diabetes. Now, that's a win, no matter how you slice it.

Don't get me wrong: I'm not telling you that being fat is a good thing. It's still true that a fit lean person (notice I said lean, not thin) is still healthier overall than a fit overweight person. However, in the grand scheme of things, fitness has more benefits. According to studies from the Cooper Institute in Dallas, fitness is downright lifesaving. In one Cooper study of 25,000 men, the risk of premature death for obese fit men was only a third of that for unfit obese men.

It's important for sistas, in particular, to understand the value of fitness because we have some built-in genetic disadvantages that require us to take a proactive stance about keeping ourselves healthy. We must understand that there are real reasons, both genetic and cultural, that we gain more weight and keep it on longer when compared to women of other races. And then we must use that information to strengthen our commitment to a healthier lifestyle.

Dr. Ro's Walking Workout

Okay, so mountain climbing or running the marathon isn't your thing. Did you know that you can lower your blood cholesterol level by 10 points just by walking for an hour five days a week? Or that you have an equal chance of lowering your blood pressure by 10 points by walking that same hour? Now, I am a walker. My guardian, Rosetta, used to take me on long walks in the neighborhood to "see pretty birds and to smell the beautiful flowers." We'd go on long jaunts to take in a little nature. As a 12-year-old, I found it boring, and I wanted no part of this "exercise." As an adult, I find myself stopping at any chance I'm given to take in nature, just the way Rosetta taught me, and today I live for it.

Now I get up each morning and walk-jog three and a half miles. It is, to put it simply, one of the best overall exercises you can do. You get results, gradually. You can do it effortlessly, and anybody can do it. But to be honest with you, I didn't start my journey to good health waking up in the morning, raring to go out walking. And frankly, even now I find it monotonous and boring, covering the same ground on a treadmill day after day. But if you don't move your butt, the most unfortunate thing you will have done is kill yourself prematurely.

Walking works most of your largest muscles and your cardiovascular system. You use a lot of calories, burn abdominal fat, and tone your leg muscles. And if all of these benefits aren't enough, walking is the black woman's favorite word: free. You don't have to buy special equipment or clothing (except a decent pair of walking shoes to protect yourself from foot injuries and muscle and tendon strains). In addition, walking doesn't require that you set aside a lot of additional time to fit in a workout. You can just walk out of your front door and start doing it. If the weather is too cold, wet, or hot for you to enjoy an outdoor walk, you can go to a mall. Lots of malls open up in the early morning hours to accommodate walkers. Or you can go to a gym and walk on an indoor track or treadmill if you prefer. Some of you may even be fortunate enough to have such equipment at work or at home.

As you get in better shape, you'll need to increase your intensity in order to continue seeing benefits.

There are a few ways to add intensity to your walking workout: (1) walk faster, (2) walk uphill, or (3) add walking poles. Walking faster is good until you progress to the point—probably at four to four and a half miles per hour—that you can't intensify the exercise without breaking into a jog or a run. Some people wear wrist weights to maximize their walking workouts, but I don't recommend them because they can cause joint problems by throwing off your stride. The safest way to add intensity, in my experience, is by walking uphill. If you add walking poles, which resemble ski poles and can be purchased at most sporting goods stores, and which work a number of muscle groups all at once, you can burn up to 22 percent more calories than you would walking without poles, for a boost in calorie-burning potential of as much as 100 calories per hour. See Secret 10 for more ideas about my walking workout.

Many of you may choose to go beyond the walking workout and join the millions of people who enjoy jogging or running. If you do choose this more active form of exercise, keep in mind that it is harder on the joints and sometimes causes muscle sprains, so be sure to warm up gradually for five minutes and then stretch. Also, if you've only recently begun to exercise, build up to running or jogging with at least 10 weeks of aerobic activity.

The Sparks Theory

The American College of Sports Medicine (ACSM) recommends that adults get 20 to 60 minutes of aerobic exercise three to five days a week. On top of that, they say you should do two or three days of strength and flexibility training to achieve real fitness. But let's get real: Even the ACSM concedes that only about 15 percent of Americans actually do that. As for us, we're so far down on the activity scale, we barely amount to a blip on the fitness screen when sizing up our exercise commitment. So this next finding should really float your boat! Did you know that now ACSM scientists have found that you can boost your fitness status by engaging in 10-minute bouts of exercise? Eureka!

It turns out a daily half-hour workout can be broken up into 10-minute segments. Here's what the science says: 40 formerly sedentary study participants performed 10-minute "sparks" of exercise 15 times a week—in other words, just two per day for six days, and three on the seventh day. They performed 7 to 10 aerobic sparks in the form of dancing, a walk to the corner store to pick up the morning paper, or climbing stairs in their office building at lunch. They did two to four strength-training sparks by performing some sort of calisthenics or resistance exercise using weights. Then they performed flexibility sparks, such as stretching at work or at home.

When these exercise "sparks" were combined with a sensible eating plan, guess what happened? On the average, these 40 sedentary people lost three pounds in three weeks (don't laugh, that's the recommended safe weight loss, a pound a week). They boosted their aerobic capacity by 15 percent, showed strength and muscular endurance increases that ranged from 40 to 100 percent, and improved their flexibility. And here's a benefit you can take home to Mama: They reduced their cholesterol level by as much as 34 points. That's nothing to thumb your nose at. So what's the moral of the story? Even small amounts of exercise that seem almost effortless can make a difference in your quality of life. And this isn't the only scientific evidence that supports the small-bouts-of-exercise notion. *Circulation*, the American Heart Association's journal, published a study indicating that two 15-minute aerobic exercise sessions can curb heart disease risk as much as a 30-minute session. So if time is of the essence, and for most of us it is, this is a workable solution to your getting-fit problem.

Still think the concept of getting moving is an all-or-nothing proposition? Think again. Gone are the days when you think about moving toward good health as either a trip to the gym to work out for 30 minutes or doing nothing at all. I'm here to tell you your options are so many, you can't even wrap your beautiful head around them. We are so sedentary that adding even small amounts of activity to our days can add years to our lives. The health boost is almost immeasurable. Here is just a sampling of the benefits to you sedentary sistas:

- ❖ Reduced risk of heart disease, diabetes, colon cancer, osteoporosis (no, it's not just for our white sistas anymore), obesity, depression, and anxiety
- ❖ Improved sleep
- ❖ Greater ability to function in our daily lives

❖ Fewer aches and pains
❖ Better weight control (hallelujah)

Workin' It Out with Everyday Livin'

I can't tell you the number of times I've counseled people about the thing they just can't seem to put their finger on that makes them sad. Their spirits don't sing, and they don't see the sunshine, the flowers, and the beauty of life, all because they carry around extra weight. But they just can't seem to get to the point of doing anything about it.

But what would you say if I told you it was possible to burn 53 calories with a half hour of passionate love-making with your beloved? You could burn 35 calories just by kissing for that same half hour. I agree, a burn rate of 70 or 106 calories per hour isn't much, especially if you've just eaten 300 calories of some high-fat snack. It's probably not even double your BMR—the rate at which you burn calories at rest. But you've got to admit, boisterous sex beats the treadmill any day of the week, and you've got to start someplace!

In a Mayo Clinic study researchers found that some people, regardless of what they eat, don't gain weight as others do because they expend energy doing everyday things, like fidgeting unconsciously. While you might not be one of those "lucky" fidgety folks, if you can expend energy doing the things you like doing (such as making out with your sweetie), getting yourself moving won't be such a chore—and you're more likely to stick with it.

Sex isn't the only non-gym-related calorie burner.

Do you enjoy gardening, tossing a Frisbee with your children, walking your dog, ice-skating, dancing every Friday night? Guess what? You're burning calories.

Try these no-workout calorie burners and get some life. (These figures are based on a half hour of moderate movement for a woman who weighs 150 pounds. If you weigh more, you'll burn more calories; if you weigh less, you'll burn fewer calories.)

Calorie-Burning Hobbies

Easy bike riding (11 mph)	210 calories
Fast dancing	193 calories
Slow dancing	105 calories
Playing drums	140 calories
Riding horseback	91 calories

Calorie Burners Around the House

Bringing in firewood	335 calories
Chopping firewood	175 calories
Stacking firewood	188 calories
Gardening (planting and weeding)	150 calories
Mowing the lawn (with push mower)	200 calories
Tree pruning with hand saw	238 calories
Raking leaves	135 calories
Shoveling snow	300 calories
Trimming hedges with manual clippers	163 calories
Washing or waxing the car	112 calories

Calorie Burners to Do with the Kids

Playing in the snow	175 calories
Dodgeball or hopscotch	175 calories
Throwing a Frisbee	105 calories
Playing kickball	245 calories
Jumping rope	280 calories
Roller-skating	245 calories
Flying a kite	105 calories
Pushing your bundle of joy in a stroller	88 calories
Coaching your daughter's soccer team	140 calories

Putting Food and Fitness in Perspective

Although it's nice to know that we can burn calories just by doing activities that we actually enjoy, let's put some of this in perspective by comparing calories burned in these ways with the calories consumed when you put certain foods in your mouth. For example, if you eat an order of Burger King French Toast Sticks, you'd have to play kickball for an hour to burn them off. Or maybe you're feeling like a little cinnamon, so you stop by the Einstein Brothers bagel shop for a 4-ounce cinnamon bagel. You'd have to ride a horse for two hours. Feel like a little Coca-Cola? An 8-ounce glass will cost you 20 minutes of jumping rope. Riding horseback and playing kickball are ways to get some fun and fitness in your life. So if these are motivators to get you moving, I say go for it.

The Benefits of Muscle

Since muscle is a tissue that burns more calories than fat does, it is worth building more muscle to get a better, more effectively running "engine." Now, I know what you're thinking: "I don't want to look like a guy." I've heard this little quip far too many times. Believing that strength training will make you a hard-bodied man is myth number one. Actually, you'd have to work that body overtime and then supplement with some pretty hard stuff to get the pecs of body builders. And you'd have to change your eating habits drastically to see that kind of change in your body. In other words, just by virtue of your womanly body structure, you have nothing to worry about.

But here's something you might want to consider. If you've been on the diet seesaw, losing and gaining the equivalent of several Mack trucks for most of your adult life, you have probably reduced your BMR. Fad diets and drastic caloric restriction do cause weight loss, but scientists have discovered that when we diet, 25 percent of what we lose is water, muscle, bone, and lean tissue—*not* fat. By reducing your muscle mass through dieting, you have lowered your metabolism. That's why it's so easy to gain the weight back after you resume your normal eating habits. Being a part of the yo-yo diet set and habitually dieting can permanently lower your metabolic rate. That means you may be burning as much as 500 to 1,000 fewer calories than normal.

For these reasons and more, I strongly recommend strength training. Much has been written about the benefits of cardiovascular training. But until recently, little attention had been given to strength training, an important component of a balanced fitness program. A well-designed strength-training program can provide the following benefits:

✤ Increased strength of bones, muscles, and connective tissue (the tendons and ligaments), which decreases the risk of injury.
✤ Increased muscle mass. Most adults lose about one-half pound of muscle per year after the age of 20. This is largely due to decreased activity. Since muscle tissue is a good calorie burner, BMR increases as muscle mass increases, making it easier to maintain a healthy body weight.
✤ Increased weight loss.
✤ Enhanced quality of life. As general strength increases, the effort required to perform daily routines (carrying groceries, working in the garden) will be less taxing.
✤ Reduced risk of osteoporosis.

Don't worry—if you don't have the funds for a gym membership, you can strength-train at home. All you need is a space large enough for a chair and a set of dumbbells (they come in 3-, 5-, 6-, 8-, and 10-pound increments; if you need to start with lighter weights, substitute 1-pound cans of food for dumbbells). Then start slowly. One set of 8 to 12 repetitions, working the muscle to the point of fatigue, is usually sufficient. Breathe normally throughout the exercise. Lower the weight with a slow, controlled motion throughout the full range of motion. Lifting the weight to a count of two and lowering it to a count of three or four is effective. When you are able to perform 12 repetitions of an exercise correctly (without cheating) and easily, it's time to move up to heavier weights. For more information on how to do a home strength-training workout, see Dr. Miriam Nelson's books *Strong Women Stay Slim* and *Strong Women Stay Young.*

Even though I must sometimes fight the urge to lie in bed instead of doing my exercise regimen, I try to walk four to five times a week and train with free weights for 30–45 minutes at least three times a week. This routine has become as regular a part of my daily life as brushing my teeth—and just as important, if not more, to my quality of life.

Keeping Track: The Journal Approach

One way to know exactly how well you're doing on your exercise goals is to write them down and then keep track of what you did each day to meet them. Maybe your goal is just to walk the three flights of stairs to your apartment when you get home each night from work and walk a mile at the mall on Saturday and Sunday. If you've been completely inactive for years, that may seem ambitious enough. Or maybe you've been walking a mile every day for years and have decided it's time to add a half hour of strength training twice a week to this regimen. Whatever your goal, write it down and then keep a daily diary of your activities. And keep upping your goals over time. You may be surprised to find that you want to, because the rewards in how you feel and how you look will make it seem so worthwhile.

Now that you understand a little more about how your body works and how it benefits from having a healthier lifestyle, we'll start to get to the "meat" of the matter—the food choices you should be making as part of that lifestyle. As you move on through the book, we'll talk about diets, popular myths and misconceptions, and how to use them to your benefit.

Frequently Asked Questions

Q   Dr. Ro: I have relatives on both sides of my family with diabetes. Is diabetes hereditary?

A   *Type I and type II diabetes both seem to have a genetic component, but in neither form is there any absolute way of determining whether or not you are going to get it, because a whole host of other factors come into play, including (as discussed earlier) your lifestyle choices—diet and exercise—as well as possible environmental triggers that still need to be identified with certainty. There is definitely a link between genetics and type I diabetes, but the actual identity of the problem gene is not known. And the link is relatively weak compared to type II. By some estimates, if both your parents have type I diabetes, the chances are somewhere between 1 in 10 and 1 in 4 that you will develop it, whereas if both your parents have type II diabetes, you have a 1 in 2 risk. If your identical twin develops type I diabetes, you have about a 50 percent chance of developing it, too, whereas if your identical twin develops type II, you have about a 75 percent risk. With type II diabetes there is also a racial component to the genetics of diabetes, for certain ethnic groups, among them those of African descent, are prone to this form of diabetes— perhaps in our case because of that thrifty gene we discussed earlier. But genetically caused diabetes is almost certainly more the exception than the rule, and most of the people who are involved in the current epidemic of type II diabetes that is sweeping this country should probably put the blame on their diet and exercise choices rather than on their parents or grandparents.*

It has been shown that people who live in areas that have not become westernized in their diet habits (eating too much fat, too few whole grains, and too little fiber) and their exercise habits (living a sedentary lifestyle) do not get type II diabetes, no matter how high their genetic risk. The major associated risk factor for diabetes is obesity, particularly the type where you carry most of your fat around your waist. And even if you have both racial and genetic tendencies toward diabetes, studies indicate that modest weight loss, about 5 to 7 percent of body weight, and regular exercise can at least delay, if not altogether prevent, the onset of diabetes. So if one or both of your parents has type II diabetes, you and your siblings should be especially vigilant about diet and exercise in order to offset the increased risk for developing the disease. Discuss appropriate screening, lifestyle interventions, and treatment with your physician.

Q Dr. Ro: I just had a baby, and the weight I gained during my pregnancy won't go anywhere! I used to be a size 10, I'm twenty-something, and after two small girls, I'm feeling doomed! What can I do? Their father won't encourage me to exercise; he doesn't care enough. Please give me the quick fix to happiness!

A *My sista-friend, we'll start with your seemingly low self-esteem. This is a tough pill, but I must insist that you take your medicine. You've got to care enough about yourself (and those girls) to get fit without depending on encouragement from others. Frankly, those girls should be enough to get you moving. If you're not in good shape for them, then for whom will you get in shape? They'll need you for many years to come. Sure, it would be nice to have the man in your life be on board with your fitness picture, because fitness is a family affair. However, it's your size, your heart, and your other muscles and limbs at stake. And you alone are responsible for them.*

For starters, thank the Creator for your pint-size motivators. Kids are energy-filled machines that require you to be in good shape in order to keep up with them. But don't take their energy for granted. According to the American Council on Exercise, only 37 percent of American children are physically active by the time they reach high school. So setting a good example for the little ones now will protect them later. The side benefit is that you get in shape at the same time. Here's how to begin. If you don't already have them, get bikes for the family (they don't have to be new). Go on nature walks with the family and teach the kids about flowers, birds, bugs, and trees; step up the pace for a better calorie burn. Get your kids' help doing yard work, gardening, and other work around the house. By all means, get out of the house on the weekends, and use it for quality family time to get moving!

Note for would-be moms: Be advised that working out before and during the pregnancy will help you and your baby in the long run. Pre-pregnancy fitness is of crucial importance in the successful delivery of your baby and helps you to get back into shape much quicker than a mom who's unfit. Once your bouncing bundle of joy has arrived, take her to the playground, do lunges with her in the stroller, and walk, walk, walk. Do a reliable and enjoyable form of cardio at least four times a week.

Q Dr. Ro: Why can't I just take a pill for my high blood pressure? Why do I need to change my diet and start exercising?

A Although there is a wide variety of effective medicines to treat hypertension, virtually all of them cause side effects and pose potential problems when used with other drugs because of drug interactions. These problems can be amplified by the frequent need for long-term treatment. And the side effects (lethargy, headache, edema, sexual dysfunction, persistent cough) often reduce patient compliance. Nearly every black family has a hypertensive member who refuses to take her blood pressure medication because she dislikes the way it makes her feel. Lifestyle changes have no such negative side effects and can often do as much to reduce the risk of a cardiovascular event such as heart attack or stroke as medications.

So before you are forced to go on a drug to keep your blood pressure down, try to prevent the need for medication with these lifestyle changes:

- ✣ Keep body weight within 15 percent of your ideal.
- ✣ Limit daily salt intake to less than 2,400 mg—or better yet, less than 1500 mg.
- ✣ Maintain adequate dietary intake of potassium, calcium, and magnesium.
- ✣ Reduce intake of saturated fat and cholesterol.
- ✣ Do an aerobic exercise (i.e., walking, swimming, cycling) at least three times a week, aiming for a heart rate in your aerobic training zone range.
- ✣ Limit daily alcohol intake to a maximum of 24 ounces of beer, 8 ounces of wine, or 2 ounces of liquor.
- ✣ Quit smoking.

Of course, if your blood pressure is dangerously high and your doctor feels you need to get it under control immediately, take the pills—and also take the above advice. Eventually you may be able to wean yourself off the medication.

Q   Dr. Ro: I don't mind walking, but I get to the point when nothing seems to work anymore, and then I get disappointed and frustrated. What do I do to keep fit and to stick to my plan?

A   *On any workout plan there's a good chance that you'll hit the brick wall after repeating the same drill for a while. In other words, plateaus are par for the course. Not to worry. If you step up your routine by changing one or two things from time to time, you will begin to see a difference. Simple changes such as adding varying speeds and or lengths of time walking at various intervals will help more than you may think. Try warming up for 5 minutes, then walk at a comfortable pace for the next 5 minutes. Step it up by walking faster for the next 5 minutes. Then slow down your pace for the next 10 minutes. Speed it up for 5 minutes more. Finally, cool down for the final 5 minutes. That makes 35 minutes of walking at various paces. You can also try adding hills and inclines, or equipment such as walking poles that burn calories and work more muscle groups as you walk. Don't forget to add a weight- or strength-training routine to your daily workout, and watch the results that will come.*

Q   Dr. Ro: Do I get the same benefit from walking in a leisurely manner that I would get if I walked faster? What's the difference to my physical fitness?

A   A 150-pound woman who walks three miles per hour for 30 minutes burns 119 calories. That same woman covering the same amount of ground at four and a half miles per hour would burn 153 calories. Brisk walking at a pace that makes it hard for you to carry on a conversation with a walking partner is the better way to lose weight and to achieve physical fitness at a much quicker pace. For one, you burn more calories and cover more ground, but most important, you work more muscle groups. Brisk walking is of greater benefit to your physical fitness because you can burn almost as many calories as you would if you were jogging, yet you do it without the added stress on the knees, joints, and your whole body. Be sure you keep up good posture—if not, you could blow your whole plan. Bend those elbows at a 90-degree angle and keep them close to your body. Swing those arms so that on the downswing they practically brush your hips. As you move forward, swing your arms upward so that your hands are level with your breastbone.

Secret 3

Food Can Save Your Life

 It has become a daily occurrence: scientists and researchers announcing the latest findings about how our eating habits can impact our health. You've probably heard snippets on the news about how the vitamin E in almonds, spinach, and wheat germ may help prevent Alzheimer's disease, how black raspberries have the ability to fight colon cancer, how the lycopene in cooked tomatoes can prevent cancer, and how omega-3 fatty acids—found in salmon, swordfish, and tuna—can help relieve depression, premenstrual syndrome, and even attention deficit disorder.

The truth is that regardless of whether these specific claims turn out to be true, eating well is good for you in a number of ways. It can help you to lose weight if you need to, pump up your energy levels, and increase your overall sense of well-being, not to mention decrease your risk of developing illnesses, especially the ones from which black folks suffer disproportionately, including diabetes, cancer, heart disease, and stroke. And healthful eating habits, in combination with physical activity, can help you look a lot better, too—not just your figure but your hair, skin, and fingernails.

The best way to get these nutritional benefits is from real foods, because real foods are rich in antioxidants and phytochemicals—big words to describe chemical compounds that work to protect you from disease.

Key components in the antioxidant and phytochemical world are fruits and vegetables, which supply the majority of the essential vitamins and minerals we need to live. They taste great, are low in calories, and can reduce your risk of contracting many diseases. They are an important energy source, and they aid in digestion. Yet only 25 percent of people in this country eat the five to nine daily servings recommended by the USDA Food Guide Pyramid.

Phytochemicals

Phytochemicals are naturally occurring compounds in plants. Many of them have been shown to protect us against heart disease, cancer, and other chronic diseases associated with aging. There are many thousands of phytochemicals we already know about, and probably many thousands more still to be discovered. Organized into such basic groupings as carotenoids, flavonoids, isoflavones, and allylic sulfides, they are found in fruits, vegetables, nuts, legumes, and grains.

You've probably read some of the popular press

reports on a few of these phytochemicals, like the lycopene in tomatoes and the lutein in dark green leafy vegetables—both of which come under the category of carotenoids. Or maybe you've heard something about the isoflavones, the phytoestrogenic components found in particularly high quantities in soy as well as in lower amounts in dried beans. The isoflavones in soy protein help strengthen bones, specifically the bones of the spine, as well as help control hot flashes. That's great news for those of you in menopause.

Antioxidants

So why do we need antioxidants? The short answer is that they fight free radicals, which damage the cells and tissues of your body. Free radicals are unstable molecules formed as part of the body's normal metabolic processes when the cells use oxygen to produce energy. They are unstable because they are missing an electron. Once the free radicals form, they attempt to become stable by attaching to electrons from other molecules, causing those molecules to become unstable in turn. This sparks a chain reaction that can cause major cell damage and lead to life-threatening diseases. Antioxidants stop this process because they don't become unstable when a free radical steals one of their electrons. Instead, they act as a built-in repair system, bringing stability to instability. You can think of them as the body's natural protection against the aging and disease processes caused by free radicals.

Though our bodies have a natural supply of antioxidants, they are not enough.

Plant-based antioxidants—such as those found in beta-carotene, alpha-carotene, and vitamins C and E—consumed in a diet rich in fruits and vegetables help augment our bodies' natural antioxidants. So it's important to eat plenty of veggies and fruits in order to help ward off disease and the problems associated with aging. As it happens, many of the foods that are richest in antioxidants are also richest in phytochemicals.

Fiber

Fiber is the part of fruits, vegetables, and legumes (beans and peas) that you can't digest, and it is an absolutely crucial part of the diet. Which may sound totally illogical, but isn't. So how could something you can't digest be so important? There are two types of fiber: *insoluble fiber*, the kind found in whole-grain products and many fruits and vegetables, which passes through the intestines without being broken down and cleans them out along the way, and *soluble fiber*, the soft, sticky type found in oats, dried peas and beans, and the skins of apples, which lowers blood cholesterol levels by binding to fatty substances and moving them out of your body. You might remember that there was a time when high-fiber diets were all the rage, because studies of Bantu peoples in South Africa seemed to show that their high-fiber way of eating was the factor that was responsible for their extremely low colon cancer rates. But when other studies, including 16 years' worth of follow-up among women in the Nurses' Health Study, did not support that conclusion, suddenly fiber was out.

But fiber should be in again, because even if it doesn't prevent colon cancer, it offers a lot of other benefits to your gastrointestinal tract. If you start eating more fruits, vegetables, and legumes, you can throw away those laxatives you've been taking, because you won't have constipation anymore. And you'll also be helping to prevent conditions such as diverticulosis, diverticulitis, and irritable bowel syndrome.

For those of you who want to lose weight, fiber is a great appetite suppressant because it fills you up faster and keeps you feeling full longer, thanks both to its bulk and to the fact that it delays the absorption of food. The fact that it slows the absorption of food also means that it makes your blood sugar and insulin levels more stable, which can help to prevent or alleviate type II diabetes. When you think about all those benefits, and add to them fiber's ability to lower cholesterol, which helps lower heart disease risk, you can see why I think fiber deserves a lot more good press than it has received in recent years.

Beans, Beans, Good for (More than) Your Heart

More great news: A recent study points out that the isoflavones in soybeans (and in lesser quantities in dried beans) play a key role in the chemical process that keeps your arteries supple. Bean eaters had higher levels of these isoflavones than women who didn't eat beans regularly. Then there's the recent study that found that women who ate these legumes at least four times a week had a 22 percent lower risk of heart disease than those who had a once-a-week habit. Beans help to protect you from heart disease in part because of the natural soluble fiber they contain, which, as pointed out above, has a cholesterol-lowering effect. An added benefit of eating more beans (I recommend no less than ½ cup a day) is that it helps you to avoid high-fat, high-calorie foods; as noted in the last section, the fiber in beans gives you a feeling of fullness. By staving off hunger and making snacking between meals or overeating at meals less of a temptation, this feeling of fullness is one of your best weapons in the fight against overweight and obesity. Unfortunately, research shows that U.S. diets are relatively low in fiber, with most adults eating only half the recommended daily amount of 30 grams. Contrast this country's eating habits with those of folks in Kenya, Uganda, and Malawi, where 80 to 90 grams of fiber are eaten daily. Less than 15 percent of these countries' citizens are overweight or obese, while we suffer from an overweight and obesity rate of 61 percent. In general, obesity is rare in populations that consume high-fiber diets.

Beyond Beans

But beans aren't even the tip of the iceberg. There are so many other foods you should be adding to your diet. Just consider some of the following findings: Flaxseed is rich in lignans, which are another form of phytoestrogens, and lignans have been shown to have powerful breast-cancer-fighting properties. At the 2000 San Antonio Breast Cancer Symposium, evidence was presented documenting that lignans slow tumor growth effectively. So add a few tablespoons of ground flaxseed to your cereal or your soy drink in the morning. And if one in eight women will develop breast cancer in their lifetime, how encouraging it is to learn that scientists at the U.S. Department of Agriculture have found a way of preventing breast cancer in rats with a new soy-modified whey protein. A soy drink with added flaxseed may help to fight breast cancer in more ways than one.

New findings suggest that foods high in vitamin C, in combination with 500 milligrams of vitamin C supplements each day, may reduce your risk of cataracts. Scientists at the University of California, San Francisco, have found that women who had higher levels of vitamin C were less likely to suffer gallbladder disease. And lycopene, found in tomatoes, red grapefruit, watermelon, and guava, is a carotenoid that has been linked with lower rates of cancer.

Carrots, dangled invitingly in front of us because they are believed to help to ward off certain eye diseases, also contain ingredients that protect against heart disease and some cancers. Onions contain compounds that lower cholesterol and prevent hardening of the arteries. Macadamia nuts are effective at lowering LDL (bad) cholesterol. Caviar—which contains the all-important omega-3 fatty acids already known to protect against heart disease—also provides protection against menstrual cramps and bipolar depression. Now, I know most of you are not likely to use caviar to deal with cramps or depression, but as you'll find out below, there are low-cost everyday foods that fight heart disease, stress, memory loss, osteoporosis, aging, and toothaches.

And by color-coding food—decreasing brown foods and adding green ones—women can fight off fibroids, the very common uterine growths that cause pelvic pain, infertility, and anemia in about 40 percent of 40-year-old women. Add reds, purples, oranges, yellows, and greens to replace brown and beige foods, and add years to your life. You can learn more about what foods can do for you in Table 3-2, which is all about the disease fighters available to us in the foods we eat—or *should* eat!

The Secret of Whole Grains

Yes, the Food Guide Pyramid tells you to include 6 to 11 daily servings of grains in your diet. What the guide doesn't tell you, however, is to be sure most of those grains are *whole* grains. From the bagel you had for breakfast to the croissant in the sandwich you had at lunch to the roll you included with dinner, most of the starches you've been scarfing down are probably made from refined, not whole, grains. That means they've been stripped of the bran and germ, which contain most of the important nutrients (fiber, lignans, antioxidants, selenium, iron, zinc), which provide protection against illness. You've been eating (gasp!) white bread, or its equivalent, and a whole lot of it.

What's the problem, you ask, with white bread? Besides the fact that it is lacking in so many important nutrients, a diet high in refined carbohydrates—such as bagels, croissants, and almost all dinner rolls, not to mention biscuits, white rice, most muffins, and that pretzel you ate for your afternoon snack—is quick to raise blood sugar in your body, and that is something African Americans need to be particularly careful about because of our tendency toward insulin resistance, syndrome X, and type II diabetes. As we learned in Secret 2, syndrome X is a condition in which the body makes more insulin than necessary after the consumption of carbohydrates—especially when the carbohydrates are simple, as in the case of all the sweets we eat, or refined, as in the case of the white bread and its variations. With syndrome X comes elevated blood pressure and triglycerides, which means that a diet high in sugars and refined starches could be detrimental in any number of ways.

A diet high in whole grains, however, can make a significant difference in your risk of several diseases:

♣ *Diabetes.* The landmark Nurses' Health Study found that the nurses who ate the most sugars and refined carbohydrates and the least whole grains had a two and a half times greater risk of developing type II diabetes. Those who ate the most whole grains (7.5 grams per day—which is the equivalent of a bowl of oatmeal and two slices of whole-wheat bread) were 30 percent less likely to develop type II diabetes. Recent studies show that whole grains keep your blood sugar on track, reducing your risk of developing diabetes.

♣ *Heart disease.* Two or more servings per day of whole grains lower your risk of death from heart disease

Whole Grains: Don't Be Fooled

Just because it's brown doesn't mean it should stick around. Even when you find bread that is dark in color as in the case of pumpernickel and rye, don't be fooled. Unless the ingredients panel lists whole grain ingredients on the label, and lists those ingredients first, the color is meaningless.

Annette Lee, the mother of a friend and colleague of mine, suffered from mild high blood pressure, and her husband had been diagnosed with type II diabetes. Both diseases, plus breast cancer and heart disease, run rampant in her immediate and extended families. And since hitting menopause, she'd packed on more than a few extra pounds. Determined to take control of their health, the couple made dietary changes, including switching from white to stone-ground wheat bread, and started walking three times a week. They thought they were on the right track, and with their walking program they were. But what they didn't know was that the bread they'd been eating wasn't whole-wheat bread at all.

"I didn't know that the stone-ground wheat bread we had been buying all this time was basically white bread until a conversation with my daughter, who's a health reporter," Annette says. Now, sistas, I'm telling you: When you buy bread, check the first ingredient

continued

on the list. If the word *whole* doesn't appear, that brand is made of all or mostly refined flour. Bottom line? Don't be fooled by the color of the bread. Dark brown breads like pumpernickel aren't necessarily made from whole grains; the color in pumpernickel can come from molasses or even artificial color. So— just because it's brown, doesn't mean it should stick around.

by 30 percent. One study in the *American Journal of Clinical Nutrition* found that women who eat three servings of whole grains a day have half the risk of developing heart disease compared to women who eat only refined grains.

❖ *Breast cancer.* A recent Italian study found that women who suffer from breast cancer ate more cereals, cakes, and bread made of refined grains. Diets high in whole grains have been linked to lower rates of the disease.

❖ *Colon cancer.* Chronic constipation has recently been linked to an increased risk of colon cancer. Diets high in whole grains help prevent constipation. And one study of people who ate lots of whole grains found that they had half as much colon cancer as people who ate few or no whole grains.

❖ Other studies suggest that the protective effects of whole grains against heart disease are more significant in overweight women than they are in lean women.

Dozens of recent studies have shown that, in addition to the diseases listed above, diets high in whole grains also reduce the risk of gallbladder, mouth, ovarian, and stomach cancers.

Check out the following chart to make sure you don't make the same mistake Annette made when choosing grain products.

More good news: Whole grains can also aid in your weight loss efforts. One study found that participants who ate 18 to 36 grams of whole grains daily absorbed 130 fewer calories each day. That's a potential 13-pound loss over a 12-month period.

Table 3-1 Whole-Grain Camouflage

Not Whole-Grain	Whole-Grain
Enriched flour	Brown rice
Unbleached wheat flour	Bulgur
Unbromated wheat flour	Graham flour
Enriched wheat flour	Whole-grain corn
Stone-ground wheat	Whole-wheat flour
Multigrain	Pearl barley
Seven-grain	Popcorn

Broccoli Gets Its Due

Though many adults—and their children—turn up their noses when it comes to broccoli, this much-maligned vegetable may finally be getting its props. Why? The news that it's a nutritional powerhouse has helped. Broccoli is rich in potassium, vitamin A, and vitamin C, as well as antioxidants that may help ward off cancer. It boasts a fistful of phytochemicals, including sulforaphane and indole-3-carbinol, which may detoxify cancer-causing substances before they have a chance to wreak havoc on your body. In women, indole-3-carbinol may render the estrogen associated with breast cancer into a more benign form. And a number of studies have linked regular consumption of cruciferous vegetables—vegetables in the cabbage family, which get their name from their four-petaled flowers, which resemble a cross—to a reduced risk of breast, colon, and stomach cancers. This vegetable family includes broccoli, cauliflower, cabbage, brussels sprouts, collards, kale, mustard greens, rutabagas, turnips and turnip greens, and more.

The Nutty Connection

Nuts, though loaded with fat and often with salt, do provide health benefits. That's because the types of fat found in nuts—monounsaturated and polyunsaturated—are the good kinds of fat. Current scientific thinking suggests that a smart way to snack is to eat nuts instead of junk food high in saturated fats (like potato chips and doughnuts). That way you'll lower your blood levels of triglycerides and LDL (bad) cholesterol while raising HDL (good) cholesterol—and you've got the perfect formula for preventing heart disease. And here's another nutty benefit for your heart: Nuts contain vitamin E, a potent antioxidant that may help to further ward off heart disease.

Many nuts, including pecans and walnuts, also contain a phytochemical called ellagic acid. In preliminary laboratory studies, ellagic acid seems to trigger a process known as apoptosis, in which cancer cells kill themselves. In addition, nuts, along with oysters, liver, cocoa, and seeds, contain trace amounts of copper, a mineral that has been found to help ward off colon cancer. A recent landmark study found that diets containing healthy fats (nuts, peanut butter) helped people maintain long-term weight loss better than diets that eliminate fat altogether.

Since an ounce of nuts will add about 150 calories to your daily calorie intake, however, you'll have to limit yourself to a handful.

Saving Our Sistas

In Secret 2, I told you that black women are more likely to suffer from a number of chronic diseases than their white counterparts. Some of these diseases, such as fibroids, are debilitating but not deadly (though fibroids can cause blood loss, anemia, and severe pain, as well as infertility), while others, such as breast cancer, can indeed be fatal. Almost all can be linked to obesity and unhealthy lifestyles, and thus can potentially be prevented or minimized by the foods you eat.

Fibroids

Foods may be key in the treatment and prevention of fibroids. Since excessively high estrogen levels seem to play a role in fibroid development, research suggests that cutting down on red meat, which is believed to boost estrogen levels, could help. Furthermore, certain phytoestrogens (phytochemicals found in certain vegetables and fruits) are believed by many experts to help moderate the effect of estrogen in the body—enhancing estrogen if estrogen levels are too low, blocking estrogen's effects if the levels are too high. When Italian scientists analyzed the diets of over 2,300 women, they found that those who ate the most red meat and the least amount of green vegetables had a significantly higher incidence of fibroids than women who ate more vegetables and less red meat. Researchers currently believe that you can reduce your risk for developing fibroids by increasing your consumption of broccoli, asparagus, spinach, kale, romaine lettuce, and other green vegetables. I recommend 7 to 10 servings a day. But don't stop there. By all means, limit your consumption of red meat to no more than 3 ounces a day. Replace it with generous portions of soy protein for heart disease protection and, as an added benefit, reduction or elimination of menopausal symptoms.

Cassiella's Story: ✦ Cassiella Bonds, a fan of *Heart & Soul*, knows about fibroids. She, like 50 to 75 percent of African American women, discovered she had them. Though most of the medical research that exists about this condition links the cause of these benign growths to heredity, there is some evidence that hormones found in meat (including chicken) and dairy products may contribute to fibroids. Having seen a fibroid segment I did on *Heart & Soul*, 32-year-old Cassiella had already determined that she would not go under the knife, which might interfere with her ability to have children. So she eliminated meat and replaced the fatty foods in her diet with brown rice and soybeans. Three months after changing her diet, Cassiella's fibroids were undetectable, and she had discovered what many nutritionists already know: Low-fat diets that are high in beans, nuts, and leafy green vegetables may go a long way toward preventing the formation of fibroids in the first place, or stopping them from growing even after you've developed them.

Breast Cancer

There is increasing evidence that diet plays a part in breast cancer development. Though a lot of the research is conflicting, this much is clear: As much as 30 percent of breast cancer risk may be linked to the way we eat. And since U.S. black women are diagnosed at later stages and die from this disease at higher rates than white women, it is imperative that you hear me. Current research shows a possible connection between eating cured meats (hot dogs, bacon, lunch meat) or very well done or charred meat, especially beef, and an increased risk of developing breast cancer. These studies suggest that cancer-causing chemicals are formed when meat is cooked at high temperatures.

Does this mean that if we cut down on some of the bacon and barbecue we love so much and start eating a diet high in fruits and vegetables, we can prevent breast cancer? The jury is still out, but studies so far do seem to indicate that eating more green, yellow, orange, and red fruits and vegetables will reduce your risk of developing the disease. The yellow-orange and dark green vegetables seem to have the strongest link to a reduced breast cancer risk. So go ahead and load up on carrots, squash, sweet potatoes, spinach, and broccoli. Raw or cooked, they provide the same health benefits (although in the case of lycopene, the cancer-fighting nutrient is found in higher quantity in cooked tomatoes, tomato sauce, and tomato paste than in raw tomatoes).

Although we don't know exactly which of the many natural chemicals found in fruits and veggies may help combat breast cancer, some of the main contenders are the *carotenoids*, found in kale, parsley, tomatoes, and cantaloupe; *vitamin C*, in grapefruits, green peppers, and strawberries; *vitamin E*, in cilantro, blueberries, mangoes, and ripe olives; *folic acid*, in asparagus and lima beans; and *fiber*, which is in all fruits and vegetables, particularly blackberries, raspberries, canned prunes, dried figs, lima beans, and various dried beans. Researchers are also currently studying the cancer-preventing potential of flavonoids (found in berries), protease inhibitors (found in legumes), allium compounds (in garlic), and resveratrol (in grapes).

What does this mean to you? To put it quite simply, most Americans don't eat enough fruits and vegetables. In fact, studies show we need to double our intake nationwide in order to meet the minimum of the recommended five to nine daily servings. In short, sista-girl, you need to add more vegetables and fruits to your diet. Here are my easy suggestions for accomplishing this:

- ❖ Keep raw and prepared vegetables in the refrigerator for snacks.
- ❖ Add vegetables to soups, stews, casseroles, pizzas, and sandwiches.
- ❖ Substitute spinach or another dark green leafy vegetable such as watercress or arugula for iceberg lettuce in a salad.
- ❖ Eat baked sweet potatoes instead of baked white potatoes.
- ❖ Eat fruit as a snack.
- ❖ Drink 100 percent fruit or vegetable juice instead of cocktails or soda.
- ❖ Grate a carrot or pepper and add it to spaghetti sauce.

Menopausal Conditions

Here's a scenario taking place in hundreds of physicians' offices every day between women going through menopause and their doctors. The doctor writes out a prescription for estrogen pills or patches, saying these will replace the hormones the patient's body is no longer making, helping to eliminate her hot flashes and slowing her bone loss. The patient asks if the pills cause cancer. The doctor acknowledges that there is an increased risk of ovarian and breast cancer but argues that the improvement in quality of life and the benefit to her bones make it worth taking the chance.

As it happens, black women have been more skeptical than their white counterparts about the risks of using hormone replacement therapy (HRT) all along, and science now supports their skepticism. According to the most recent information available, the risks may not outweigh the benefits of taking HRT. Two major studies of postmenopausal women on hormone replacement—one from the National Cancer Initiative (NCI) and the other from the Women's Health Institute—found that women on HRT were at increased risk for ovarian cancer. In fact, postmenopausal women who used HRT for 10 or more years were at a significantly higher risk not just for ovarian cancer but for coronary heart disease, stroke, and pulmonary embolism.

When the news broke I received calls from clients I hadn't spoken to in years. They were panic-stricken and at a loss for what their options would be if they gave up their pills and patches. They had menopausal symptoms, and they wanted (dare I say, deserved) solutions.

Sistas, take heart: There are dietary steps that can make menopause much more manageable. They are better for your heart and bones than estrogen prescriptions could ever hope to be, and they accomplish these things without the side effects.

Hot Flashes: ✦ Mayan women in Yucatán, Mexico, don't report any hot flashes. Only about 10 percent of Japanese women report having hot flashes with menopause. By contrast, nearly two-thirds of Western women report having them. The difference between women in the United States, for whom hot flashes are common, and Mayans and Japanese, for whom they are rare or unknown, appears to be diet. The Mayan diet consists of corn and corn tortillas, beans, tomatoes, squash, sweet potatoes, and radishes, with very little meat, and no dairy products. The traditional Japanese diet is also extremely low in meat, dairy, and fat, while being high in soy and fish protein. The animal-based meals of the Western diet affect hormone levels and undoubtedly contribute to the menopausal problems that are common in Western countries.

Hot flashes are the external sign of internal drops in estrogen levels. The estrogen-like compounds, called phytoestrogens, found in soybeans can help offset the drop in estrogen. Studies report hot flashes can be reduced by up to 40 percent when women add soy to their diets. But how much is enough? I suggest 15 ounces of soy milk (about 2 cups) or 2 ounces of tofu daily might be all you need to help stop hot flashes. Be aware that recent studies have found a possible link between soy and breast cancer, so if you are a breast cancer survivor or at increased risk for developing the disease because of a family history, don't increase your soy intake until you speak with your physician.

Other natural ways to combat flashes include increasing vitamin E intake and reducing consumption of caffeine, alcohol, hot beverages, and spicy foods. For a good night's sleep, you might want to add the herb sage—the same sage you use to season your Sunday chicken and stuffing. There is growing evidence that including sage in the diet may ward off night sweats, another menopausal symptom. Add 4 tablespoons of dried sage to a cup of boiling water. Cover and steep as you would a tea, but let it sit for four hours before straining. Then drink before bedtime for a restful night's sleep.

Osteoporosis: ✦ One of the causes of this bone-thinning ailment is decreased estrogen after menopause. Women may lose between 2 and 5 percent of their bone mass every year for five years after going through the change of life. Their bones become more brittle and are more likely to break. In older women, hip fractures due to osteoporosis can be fatal. And contrary to popular belief, African American women do get osteoporosis. Helen Smith, who read my column in *Heart & Soul Magazine*, had a bone density test done as part of a battery of tests her physician suggested after she reached 55. She was shocked to find out she was borderline for developing osteoporosis. "I thought only small-boned women, like white women, got osteoporosis," she says. "In fact, I went to a retreat and a black nurse said black women don't get it. I thought being black myself meant that I was protected."

Sistas, you should know that you start losing bone around age 30; that's why it's important for women of all ages and races to strengthen bone mass with weight-bearing exercise like walking, running, and weight lifting and through a diet rich in calcium, phosphorous, and vitamin D. Because most African American women don't get enough calcium in their diets, I recommend taking a multivitamin that includes calcium, iron, and antioxidants. If you are taking calcium supplements, your body makes better use of the calcium when you take it with protein in the same meal. How much calcium is enough? The Recommended Dietary

Allowance (RDA) is 800 milligrams per day for women under 50 (premenopausal) and 1,000 milligrams and 1,500 milligrams for women 50 and older. But I recommend (as does the medical community) 1,200 milligrams and 1,500 milligrams, respectively. Nonfat milk or soy milk fortified with calcium and vitamin D are good sources of these nutrients (vitamin D is essential for transporting calcium into the bones). In addition to soy milk, many other soy foods are also rich in calcium. One cup of cooked soybeans contains roughly 12 percent of your daily allowance for calcium. Be mindful that some foods have substances in them that can interfere with calcium absorption in the body. The oxalates in spinach and the phytates in legumes and some whole grains, for example, bind to calcium and prevent the body from using it efficiently. So be careful to avoid eating spinach, legumes, and whole grains in the same meal as the calcium-rich foods, or at the same time that you take your calcium supplements.

Heart Disease: ✦ Your risk for heart disease escalates quickly as estrogen levels drop after menopause. Since recent reports have found hormone replacement therapy may do more harm than good when it comes to preventing postmenopausal heart disease, you'd do well to reduce your heart disease risk through diet and exercise. The Food and Drug Administration (FDA) recently approved a health claim that a diet including soy protein and low in saturated fat and cholesterol reduces heart disease risk. This claim, which can be found on the label of almost any food that contains soy protein, came as a result of a number of studies showing that 25 grams of soy protein a day could offer real benefits. Adopt a low-fat, high-fiber diet that includes a wide range of fresh fruits and vegetables, whole-grain breads and cereals, legumes (including soybeans), and nonfat dairy products. This can help you keep blood fat levels low and heart disease at bay. In addition, studies show that the sulfides found in garlic can reduce cholesterol and may make the blood less "sticky" and therefore less likely to form clots, which may provide additional protection for your heart.

Memory Loss: ✦ If you find you are having trouble remembering where you put your keys or your purse, don't panic. Many women experience memory and concentration problems during perimenopause and after menopause. Some scientists believe that you may be able to minimize these memory problems with blueberries. Pint for pint, blueberries may contain more antioxidants than any other fruit or vegetable. The most powerful health-promoting compounds in these little blueberries are anthocyanins, phytochemicals that belong to the flavonoid family—which, in addition to combating the free-radical damage that leads to heart disease, may also boost brain power. In laboratory studies, aging animals fed a blueberry-rich diet for four months performed as well in memory tests as younger animals.

Colon Cancer: ✦ Although African Americans have only a slightly higher incidence of colorectal cancer than our white counterparts, we tend to suffer a more virulent form of the disease and to have a 30 percent higher death rate from it. New research, however, suggests that calcium can reverse this trend. And among people who had low-calcium diets, even a modest increase in calcium appears to lower the risk of some types of colon cancer by about 50 percent. The calcium you need—the folks in the study got about 700 milligrams a day—should come from a food source, if possible.

Test Your Vitamin and Mineral IQ

Can guzzling orange juice really prevent the common cold? What's the best dietary source of calcium to combat osteoporosis? What's the best way to boost your mineral intake? These are just some of the many questions I get about food, supplements, and health. Find out just how vitamin and mineral savvy you really are with my vitamin and mineral quiz.

1. You're gearing up for cold and sniffle season, so you start popping a vitamin C supplement each day to keep the doctor away. Can vitamin C help prevent the common cold?
   a) Yes
   b) No

2. In which way can adults between the ages of 19 and 50 meet their daily need for calcium, the bone-strengthening mineral?
   a) eating 3 cups of broccoli
   b) eating 3 cups of spinach

     c) *eating 3 cups of nonfat yogurt or skim milk or 1½ ounces of natural cheese*

     d) *only by taking a supplement—food alone won't cut it*

3. The B vitamin folate (folic acid) may help reduce the risk of:

     a) *heart disease*

     b) *colon cancer*

     c) *certain birth defects*

     d) *all of the above*

4. Which of the following delivers the highest levels of vitamin A?

     a) *2 cups of skim milk fortified with vitamin A*

     b) *½ cup baked sweet potato*

     c) *½ cup cooked carrots*

     d) *a 2-ounce milk chocolate candy bar*

5. You want to add some vitamin E to your diet for its antioxidant properties. Which one of the following provides the greatest amount of vitamin E per serving?

     a) *2 tablespoons peanut butter*

     b) *¼ cup wheat germ*

     c) *a 6-ounce glass of tomato juice*

     d) *½ medium avocado*

6. If you're eating whole-wheat bread as part of your breakfast, what should you do to increase your body's ability to absorb the iron in the bread?

     a) *smear some jelly on the bread*

     b) *have the bread with a 4-ounce grapefruit juice chaser*

c) toast the bread

d) eat it dry

7. To preserve the vitamins in your vegetables, what is the best cooking method?

a) microwave them

b) bake them

c) steam them

d) any of the above methods will do

Responses—

1. After reviewing all the cold and sniffle research, the Institute of Medicine concluded that swallowing loads of vitamin C supplements will not prevent a person from catching a cold. However, it can decrease the length and severity of the cold in some individuals. But before you start popping vitamin C tablets, know that vitamin C is water-soluble, so taking more than your body can absorb—probably anything in excess of 1,500–3,000 milligrams—will only result in your having the most expensive urine in town. Another fact to bear in mind is that large amounts of vitamin C, if taken over long periods of time, can cause kidney stones and stomach problems such as cramps, diarrhea, and nausea. The minimum requirement for women between 15 and 60 years of age who are not pregnant or breast-feeding is 60 milligrams a day, the amount found in ¾ cup of OJ. Orange juice, anyone?

2. Three cups of broccoli would provide only 216 milligrams of calcium, about one-fourth of the 1,000 milligrams recommended daily for adults in this age group.

Don't let that discourage you from steaming up a head of this cancer-fighting powerhouse, because it's also jam-packed with other nutrients. While spinach is a fabulous source of the B vitamin folic acid, this leafy green vegetable binds the calcium that it contains so tightly that your body absorbs little of it. And while a calcium supplement is a viable way to meet your daily calcium needs, you should first try to get it from food. The best answer? A cup of yogurt, a cup of milk, or 1 to 1½ ounces of natural cheese each provides about 300 milligrams of calcium. Three servings of any of these foods will total up to about 1,000 milligrams of calcium, the amount recommended daily for adults 19 to 50 years of age.

3. The answer is all of the above. Folate may help fight heart disease and colon cancer and help reduce the risk of certain birth defects when consumed before a woman conceives and during the first several weeks of pregnancy. Not bad for one little vitamin.

4. Sweet potatoes win hands down. A modest half-cup serving of baked sweet potatoes provides slightly more than 950 micrograms of the active form of vitamin A. An adult male needs 900 micrograms of the active form of vitamin A daily, whereas nonpregnant adult females should consume 700 micrograms a day on average. Carrots are your next best bet: Eat a half cup of cooked carrots and you'll rack up more than 850 micrograms of the active form of vitamin A. So start scraping those carrots. Two cups of milk would meet more than 30 percent of an adult's daily need. But there isn't enough milk in milk chocolate to even put a dent in your needs. A 2-ounce bar of milk chocolate provides only about 30 micrograms of vitamin A and, on average, more than 300 empty calories.

5. The number one choice? A quarter cup of wheat germ provides slightly more than 20 percent of an adult's recommended daily intake of vitamin E. Start sprinkling some wheat germ on your cereal, yogurt, or fresh fruit. A hefty smear of peanut butter, preferably on a slice of whole-wheat bread, is the second highest source of vitamin E on this list. Tomato juice is the third highest in this group, providing slightly more than 10 percent of an adult's recommended daily amount of vitamin E. Try lower-sodium tomato juice on the rocks with a slice of lemon; it's an easy way to get some E. Of the foods listed here, avocado has the lowest amount, but it still provides a respectable 8 percent of an adult's recommended daily vitamin E.

6. Vitamin C enhances your body's ability to absorb the type of iron that is found in plant-based foods such as bread and grains. In fact, adding 25 milligrams of vitamin C to your meal can double the amount of iron absorbed from whole-wheat bread. A mere 4 ounces of grapefruit juice provides 36 milligrams of vitamin C. Orange juice is another super vitamin C source. Better yet—eat a grapefruit or an orange!

7. You can't go wrong. According to the USDA, about 80 to 100 percent of vitamins are preserved in most cooked vegetables whether they are steamed, microwaved, or baked, so long as you don't overcook them. The trick to avoid cooking the vitamins out of your veggies is to cook them only until tender, and in just enough

water to create steam but not so little that you'll be up to the wee hours scouring pans. If you are cooking them in a pot, use a lid that fits the pan so that the veggies will cook quickly. When it comes to cooking Mother Nature's finest, use whatever cooking method works best for you—just keep those healthy veggies coming!

Science and Healthy Eating

While we still don't know enough about what foods will do the most for us, never before has science been so willing to give food and lifestyle so much credit for disease prevention. The food industry is helping in that area, too. Did you know that soon you'll be able to walk right up to your produce section and buy broccoli that's been bred to contain three times more antioxidants to fight cancer than the stuff you've been able to get in the past? Tomatoes will contain far more beta-carotene, another cancer-fighting substance, because of genetic engineering.

Now, it's true that there is major debate over genetically modified foods (also called genetically modified organisms, or GMOs). The pros: By increasing crop production, we can provide enough food to end world hunger. We can also fight diseases and malnutrition, and increase the shelf life of many foods. The cons: Opponents of genetic modification believe we are producing unnatural foods and playing God, with health consequences that can't be predicted, and possibly dangerous effects on the environment as well. Though the jury is still out on GMOs, it is important to note that each day begins anew with discoveries, and many of them will help save lives. We shouldn't automatically reject anything new just because it's not found in nature. Instead, we should encourage research that has the potential to improve health.

In this chapter we've discussed the major health-aiding foods, but check out Table 3-2 below for a more complete list of how to beat disease through diet.

Table 3-2 Disease-Fighting Nutrients and Food Components

Beneficial Nutrients / Healing Powers	Some Foods Containing Nutrient
Anthocyanins *Phytochemicals that fight cancer and heart disease*	*Olives*
Beta-carotene *An antioxidant that improves night vision, protects against macular degeneration and heart disease, reduces cataract risk, promotes healthy skin, fights infection*	*Carrots; broccoli; red, green, and orange bell peppers; liver; sweet potatoes; cantaloupe; squash*
Calcium *Strengthens bones, prevents osteoporosis, lowers blood pressure, lowers cholesterol, fights colon polyps, fights PMS*	*Lowfat milk, cheese, and yogurt; broccoli; canned salmon with bones*

Beneficial Nutrients/ Healing Powers	Some Foods Containing Nutrient
Chromium *Helps the body to manage insulin*	*Shredded wheat, peas, corn oil*
Ellagic acid *A phytochemical that wards off heart disease, fights certain cancers*	*Berries, walnuts, pomegranates*
Fiber *Lowers cholesterol, stabilizes blood sugar, reduces cancer risk*	*Beans, berries, broccoli, wheatberries, pears, apples, oranges, apples (with skin), oatmeal, oatbran*
Flavonoids *Fight cancer and heart disease, helps to improve memory*	*Olives, blueberries, spinach, dark chocolate, oranges*
Folate *Lowers homocysteine, thereby fighting heart disease, prevents birth defects*	*Kidney beans, navy beans, pinto beans, butter beans, black beans, orange juice, spinach, asparagus*
Lutein *An antioxidant that fights macular degeneration and reduces risk of cataracts*	*Parsley, corn, squash, spinach, green leafy vegetables*

Beneficial Nutrients/ Healing Powers	Some Foods Containing Nutrient
Lycopene *An antioxidant that protects against heart disease and certain cancers*	*Tomatoes and tomato-based foods, red and pink grapefruit, watermelon*
Magnesium *Helps to fight stress, helps to prevent heart disease*	*Artichokes, spinach, wheat germ, soybeans, bananas, peanuts, oatmeal*
Niacin *Promotes healthy skin, mostly used to promote healthy enzyme function in the body and to help the body produce energy*	*Poultry, fish, beef, peanut butter, legumes, brown rice*
Omega-3 fatty acids *Prevents heart disease, fights eye disease, protects against depression and bipolar disorder*	*Salmon, walnuts, almonds, anchovies, albacore tuna, mackerel*
Polyphenols *Phytochemicals that fight cancer by inhibiting new tumor growth in blood vessels*	*Green and black teas*

Beneficial Nutrients/ Healing Powers	Some Foods Containing Nutrient
Potassium *Protects against high blood pressure, helps with muscle contraction, helps to regulate fluids and mineral balance*	*Bananas, oranges, apricots, strawberries, lowfat milk, okra, acorn squash, chickpeas, meat, poultry, fish*
Selenium *Helps to fight cancer by protecting cells, aids in cell growth*	*Seafood, organ meats such as liver and kidney, grains and seeds*
Sulforaphane *A phytochemical that fights cancer*	*Broccoli and broccoli sprouts, brussels sprouts, cabbage*
Thiamin *Helps to maintain the nervous system and may fight depression*	*Beef liver, pork, sunflower seeds, beans, fish*
Vitamin B-6 *Fights infection, helps the body to make nonessential amino acids, helps to produce hemoglobin*	*Salmon, chicken, pork, black beans, peanut butter, whole-wheat pasta, almonds*

Beneficial Nutrients/ Healing Powers	Some Foods Containing Nutrient
Vitamin C *An antioxidant that fights heart disease, some forms of cancer, and infection. Helps the body to absorb iron in plant foods such as spinach, keeps gums healthy, heals cuts and wounds*	*Oranges, orange juice, strawberries, bell peppers, tomatoes, white potatoes*
Vitamin D *Maintains bone health, necessary for the body to absorb calcium and phosphorous from milk*	*Lowfat milk, eggs, canned salmon with bones, fortified dry cereals*
Vitamin E *An antioxidant that reduces heart disease and cancer risk, may fight cataracts*	*Sunflower seeds, eggs, wheat germ, almonds, peanut butter, spinach, sweet potatoes*

Frequently Asked Questions

Q Dr. Ro: I've started taking vitamin E supplements, because I heard it's good for your heart. But I've also increased the amount of vitamin E I get through my diet. Is it possible to ingest too much vitamin E?

A *Vitamin E is found naturally in vegetable oils, nuts, seeds, leafy green vegetables, and wheat germ. I think it's safe to say that you need not worry about getting too much vitamin E through your diet. But supplements could be another matter. The Recommended Dietary Allowance (RDA) for females is 8 milligrams per day—although taking 200–800 milligrams has been considered safe. Since the labels on most supplement bottles express the amount of vitamin E in terms of international units (IU) rather than milligrams, you'll want to know that the equivalent in terms of your recommended daily vitamin E needs is 30 IU, and that studies of vitamin E toxicity indicate that a person would have to take up to 3,200 IU per day to see any consistent side effects.*

Vitamin E's primary role appears to be as an antioxidant, helping to combat free radicals—unstable molecules that attack other molecules in the body. Vitamin E may also help fight heart disease by inhibiting platelet clusters, which cause clots to form, as well as blocking the formation of thrombin, a potent hormone that also plays a role in platelet clustering.

While vitamin E is a powerful protective antioxidant, you should of course be careful not to overdose on it through the use of supplements. There are a number of circumstances under which you should not use the supplements or should do so only in consultation with your doctor. The first set of concerns has to do with its anti-clotting properties. If you are deficient in vitamin K, which helps the blood to clot, or if you are taking any doctor-prescribed anticoagulant medicines or blood thinners, you should talk to your doctor for advice about taking vitamin E supplements. Because vitamin E acts as an anticoagulant, if you take it on top of one of these medications, it could increase the risk of bleeding. Similarly, for anyone who is going to have extensive dental work or is contemplating surgery, it is advisable to stop taking vitamin E supplements well before you go under the knife so that you won't bleed or bruise excessively.

You should also be careful about using vitamin E supplements if you are taking drugs such as ulcer medications, cholesterol-lowering drugs, or an antibiotic called neomycin. Consult with your physician if you are taking these or other prescription drugs.

Q   **Dr. Ro: How many servings of fruits and vegetables do I need to eat each day to reduce my risk of breast cancer?**

A   *In the largest study of its kind, the Nurses' Health Study, researchers reported a 17 percent lower rate of breast cancer among women who consumed at least two servings per day of fruits and vegetables as compared to those who consumed less than one* serving per day. In another recent study, the consumption of more than five servings per day of vegetables versus less than three servings per day was associated with a 54 percent reduction in the breast cancer rate. The health benefits of eating fruits and vegetables have prompted the National Cancer Institute and the Produce for Better Health Foundation to co-sponsor the national "5 a Day for Better Health" program. This program is designed to encourage and provide practical ways for people to consume at least five servings per day of fruits and vegetables. However, now there is even more compelling evidence that eating 7 to 10 daily servings of fruits and vegetables, as I recommend, is even more helpful for breast cancer prevention and a number of other chronic illnesses and health problems as well.

Q Dr. Ro: I know soy is good for me, lowering my cholesterol and easing hot flashes, but I hate tofu. How can I get more soy in my diet?

A Even tofu haters love the taste and crunch of edamame, lightly cooked green soybeans. You can find them in the freezer section at large supermarkets. Just steam, peel, and eat them like peanuts. Half a cup contains 22 grams of soy protein. Other options include roasted soy nuts (a quarter cup has 19 grams of soy protein) and energy bars made with soy (GeniSoy, a leading brand, packs 14 grams of protein per bar). Another trick to try: Put firm tofu along with a little dried basil and water on pulse in your food processor (you're aiming for the consistency of ricotta cheese), then use this instead of ricotta in your lasagna. Trust me *when I say you can't tell the difference when you eat the lasagna.*

If you like smoothies, blend in soy powder (see Secret 10 for my own soy smoothie recipe). Keep in mind that the Food and Drug Administration now allows labels to note the cholesterol-lowering benefits of soy, so you'll find it easier to spot the soy burgers and other tasty items.

Q **Dr. Ro: Green tea seems to be all the rage these days, but I'm not crazy about the taste. Can I get the same health benefits from black tea?**

A *Scientists suspect that black tea, which is made from the same leaves as green tea, may be just as effective against most ailments as green tea. But green tea has been more widely studied. The health benefits of green tea are many. Studies show that green tea is the second most consumed drink in the world—water is number one—and may help strengthen bones in postmenopausal women as well as act as a powerful cancer and heart disease fighter. It is loaded with polyphenols, a class of phytochemicals with 100 times the antioxidant punch of vitamin C.*

Research suggests that one group of polyphenols in green tea, called catechins, may inhibit the growth of new blood vessels, which some scientists think may help prevent cancer by depriving early tumors of nourishment. Population studies in China link drinking green tea daily with a lowered risk of stomach, esophageal, and liver cancer. And studies from Japan show consuming 10 cups a day may reduce the risk of heart disease.

Q   **Dr. Ro: Which are better, raw vegetables or cooked ones?**

A   *That depends in part on which nutrient you're trying to get, and for what benefit. For example, a diet rich in raw vegetables can lower your risk of breast cancer, but for 37 of 48 vegetables tested, your body more easily absorbs the iron from them when they're boiled, stir-fried, steamed, or grilled. For example, the absorbable iron in cabbage jumps from 6.7 percent to 27 percent with cooking, whereby that of broccoli flowerets rose from 6 percent to 30 percent. And the lycopene in tomatoes provides the best cancer protection when the tomatoes are cooked. But let's not miss the forest for the trees. What's important is that you actually eat three to five servings or more of vegetables and two to four servings of fruit every day. However you prepare them, they're sure to do you a world of good.*

Q   **Dr. Ro: If I switch to whole grains, how many total servings of grain should I eat each day?**

A   *The Food Guide Pyramid recommends 6 to 11 daily servings of grains, but I believe this is too much, even if you eat whole grains. All grains, whether they are whole or refined, are ounce for ounce higher in calories than fruits and vegetables. A better bet is to consume three to four daily servings of grains. With that amount of food you'll get more than enough fiber to give you a feeling of fullness, which will make it less likely that you'll want to overeat.*

Secret 4

Soul Food Is Good for You!

 Now that you see that food can be a life-saver, let's examine "our food" and look at the good, the bad, and the life extension possibilities! I know the title of this secret sounds like an oxymoron; after all, you've heard from practically every health expert in the country that soul food is the stuff of which heart attacks are made.

Well, they're partly right. We put gobs of butter and high-fat cheese in our macaroni and cheese, cook collards with a hunk of fatback, and use whole milk and bacon grease in our corn bread. We fry foods in lard, salt liberally, load up on meat instead of veggies, and what veggies we do eat we cook to death. Because during slavery we couldn't afford to waste anything, we are still accustomed to finding ways to use every imaginable foodstuff, and a lot of what we find is loaded with fat. From the pig alone we get not just ham, bacon, pork chops, and roasts, but brains, neck bones, hog maws, hog jowls, ham hocks for seasoning, intestines for chitlins, fat for cracklins and lard, and hog's head, feet, and tail for souse. At every meal, whether it's a holiday or a romantic dinner for two, the table is sinking under the weight of all that food we love to serve. Remember your family's celebrations? I remember mine. There were always three or four meats (ham, fried chicken, roast beef, ribs), candied yams, potato salad, mashed potatoes, collards, pole beans, three-bean salad, macaroni and cheese, corn bread, rolls, cakes, puddings, pies. And you didn't just get two or three items and call it a day; you had to have a taste of everything, often in titanic-sized portions, with your plate piled so high you couldn't even see half of what was on it.

Why do we eat this way? Attribute it to our legacy. Certainly we may not consciously think about our ancestors when we're crafting a Thanksgiving meal from recipes handed down through the generations. But our African heritage is evident in many of the foods we prepare when we make a soul food meal, from the corn and greens to the black-eyed peas, okra, and rice, and the hard days of slavery are reflected in the determination not to let anything go to waste.

The Origin of Soul Food: From the Shores of Mother Africa to the Red Clay of the Deep South

We didn't just develop taste buds for watermelon, black-eyed peas, rice, corn, yams, and okra when the slave ships docked in North America. Many of the foods that we have come to know as our own are steeped in agricultural and culinary traditions that we brought with us all the way from West Africa. Black-eyed peas, also known as cowpeas, were eaten as staples in places like what is now Sierra Leone. There were yams in Nigeria, which were used to make a porridge-like dish called fufu, eaten with green vegetables like spinach and often mixed with stockfish—a rich, smoky, full-flavored dried fish. The yams we ate in Africa are different from the sweet potatoes found in the United States (although sweet potatoes are often mistakenly called yams here); they more closely resemble larger, rough-skinned, white-fleshed potatoes. These true yams can be traced back to Africa more than 10,000 years ago. They are native to West Africa and remain a main staple of the continent. Okra, a vegetable also indigenous to West African cooking, was used in soups, stews, and rice and vegetable dishes as a thickener, much the way it is used today, as for example in gumbo—a favorite traditional dish of the Louisiana Low Country.

Peanuts, pumpkin, even eggplant and tomatoes were also foods traditionally eaten by West Africans in their homeland, and later in this land, once the slave trade brought them here. Spices, too, were very much a part of African cuisine. Easy to grow in the rich African soil, they enabled Africa to play a significant role in the spice trade, but they were also highly valued for the aromas and flavors they added to the local cuisine. Cultural and nutritional anthropologists say Africans had a particular penchant for seasoning foods with such spices as peppercorns, ginger, cardamom, cloves, cumin, cinnamon, and turmeric. Fruits such as guava, pineapple, and papaya (known as paw-paw), nuts, seeds, vegetables, and fish—all were included in the meals eaten in our homeland.

But once in America, African slaves were forced to survive on the minimal rations granted by the slave owners. Historians say the slave owners typically gave an African family a peck of cornmeal, three pounds of bacon or salt pork, sometimes two pounds of sugar, a pound of coffee, a gallon of molasses, and some chewing tobacco, which was supposed to last for the week. They had to make the most of the meager staples available to them, so they perfected the art of stretching and improvising as they prepared food. Sometimes one chicken might have to feed a family of eight or more. Stretching meant falling back on the West African tradition of one-pot meals—cooked over fireplaces in cast-iron skillets and large kettles. Feeding their large families was possible only through a remarkable combination of resourcefulness and culinary wizardry: They obtained salt by boiling down the remains of old smokehouses, made coffee from ground okra seeds, and supplied themselves with sugar by scraping the insides of empty sugar barrels.

While the basis of the African slaves' diet was corn and pork, they supplemented that diet with fresh vegetables they grew in the small garden plots—on average less than an acre in size—allotted to them by the slave owners. There they would work on weekends, or whenever else they could find the time, trying to wrest enough sustenance from the land to keep themselves going. They planted staples such as yams and okra, which they had brought with them from their West African homeland, and they planted many other things as well: bananas, berries, pumpkins, corn, peas, kidney and lima beans, turnips, greens, and rice. Haitian slaves were also given small plots on which they were encouraged to grow food, and they added foods from their own homeland, which included mangoes, coconuts, avocados, and squash.

Historians and cultural anthropologists maintain that the deep knowledge of agriculture the Africans brought with them from the old country provided a way for them to stay connected to their ancient traditions. For thousands of years before they were taken from their homeland, they had survived on the riches of the earth. Working the land in America enabled them to remember who they were and where they had come from during the long years of their enslavement. While many of the foods the Africans ate reflected new and uncharted geographical territory, the food preparation methods they used were a continuation of the old ways—adapted, of course, to the drastic changes in circumstance brought about by slavery.

Comin' to America:
Old Foods and Traditions Get Some Soul

Both what we eat and how we prepare it reflect the long struggle to survive during the days of slavery, when our meals consisted mainly of the leftover scraps from the slave owner's meal. Somehow we managed to feed ourselves with ham hocks, chitlins, and neck bones, paired with the vegetables we grew in those small gardens, and as time passed, we combined our

African cooking traditions with flavors from the American South, and voilà! Soul Food was born.

From fish fries and barbecues to church dinners, to this day we connect with our heritage through food. For example, black folks in Chicago, Washington, D.C., and other large urban centers still preserve the tradition of frying up a batch of fish for family and friends to enjoy—just as used to be done by folks in the Deep South, from the Mississippi Delta to the Gulf Coast and beyond, back in the years before refrigeration, when the fresh catch of the day had to be celebrated and consumed immediately. Barbecues, on the other hand, can be traced back to a time when Spanish explorers in the New World met up with West Indians, who roasted meat on frames set over open fires. Adapted by the Spanish from the Arawak Indians, this method of cooking became known as *barbacoa*, meaning "to cook over coals." Historians say barbecue took center stage in all slave communities of the South. Male African slaves worked the slow-cooking hot pits—large holes in the ground lined with rocks and fueled by wood chips—which created a uniquely flavorful result. The slow cooking tenderized the meat, and the smoke from the hickory and oak chips penetrated the meat to give it a wonderful taste. Male slaves were known as the "masters of the barbecue." And to this very day, black folks still practice this art and take it very seriously.

Because soul food is both an art and a reflection of our history, it is particularly meaningful to our lives. Providing the black family with far more than mere sustenance, soul food links us to past generations and traditions, and with our brothas and sistas all across this land. Some traditional soul food cooks describe the kind of cooking they do as "vibration cooking." It's done not by measuring ingredients, but by "feeling" and sensing what they need to put in the food—a pinch of this, a touch of that, and a dash of something else. But it's also the endless amounts of love, time, and care that go into these dishes that give them their soul.

As for the methods themselves: By definition, it's not soul food if vegetables aren't mashed, creamed, candied, or simmered all day with salt pork, ham hocks, or fatback—staples of the soulful cooking art left over from the days of slavery. But while many of the recipes for soul food, whether cooked by vibration or otherwise, have been handed down from generation to generation, we modern-day African Americans who still cook this way have to recognize that we're compromising the potential nutritional benefits of the foods we have thought of as our own for hundreds of years. Our African ancestors were really on to something when they cooked collard greens, sweet potatoes, and catfish. Our traditional fare—kale, cabbage, turnip greens and other dark green leafy vegetables, red peppers, tomatoes, and watermelon, yellow and orange sweet potatoes, peppers, peaches, and carrots—are all packed with disease-fighting chemical compounds that could save our lives, as we discussed in Secret 3. It's the stuff we cook the foods with and the way we cook them that compromise their natural wholesomeness.

Soul Food Disease Fighters in Green, Orange, and Red

What have soul foods done for you lately? The obvious answer to this question is nothing, if you've been sabotaging the good works certain soul foods can do for you by cooking them badly, which I'll have more to say about below. But did you know that in their natural state—that is to say, eaten without the high-fat, high-salt foods we add to them—collard greens, for example, can protect you against cancer?

Disease-Fighting Carotenoids: The Cruciferous Vegetables

Collards, mustard greens, watercress (sometimes called "creesy salad" by down-home country folks), and kale belong to a special group of vegetables called cruciferous vegetables. Broccoli, rutabagas, brussels sprouts, turnips and turnip greens, cabbage, and cauliflower are other cousins belonging to this disease-fighting family. Cruciferous veggies contain copious amounts of phytochemicals (remember them from Secret 3?), including chemical compounds called indoles. These and other chemical compounds in the cruciferous vegetables protect us by preventing cancer cells from forming and reproducing. They may also protect us against various toxins in the environment, including cigarette smoke and air pollution, and against cataracts and macular degeneration. Gone are the days when you had to live with the prospect of getting cataracts just because it befell your grandmother. Now research has taught us that that doesn't have to be our fate. And it's all thanks to our healthful soul food preferences.

Indoles are not the only class of phytochemicals thought to be capable of preventing cancer. There are many other cancer-fighting phytochemicals, a number of which can also be found in the foods that African Americans have been eating for hundreds of years.

Disease-Fighting Carotenoids: Beta-carotene

Besides greens, another well-known staple in the African American diet is the sweet potato. Though we often eat them as candied sweet potatoes or Big Mama's sweet potato pie, dripping in butter and coated in sugar, those sweet potatoes are not just palate pleasers but potential cancer fighters, too. They contain substances called carotenoids, which are powerful antioxidants. Besides sweet potatoes, foods that are high in carotenoids include carrots and other foods with bright orange and yellow pigments. Sweet potatoes are also rich in the antioxidant vitamins A, C, and E, which help the body make white blood cells and repair the kind of cell damage that often leads to cancer as well as heart disease.

Disease-Fighting Carotenoids: Lycopene

Tomatoes are another of the cancer-fighting carotenoids in soul food fare. You may not think of them as a soul food, but during tough times black folks made sandwiches of this bright red fruit. They'd slap a couple of slices of a beefy red tomato, freshly picked from a country garden, between two slices of bread, spread mayonnaise across that bread, and call it good eatin'.

The red color in tomatoes, as in red grapefruit and watermelons (another African American favorite), comes from a carotenoid known as lycopene—an antioxidant phytochemical that seems to neutralize free radicals and help fight cancers (especially prostate cancer) as well as heart disease. Although the lycopene in watermelons is readily used by the body, a number of studies have shown that your body may have a tough time extracting the lycopene from raw tomatoes, so it seems that cooked tomatoes offer better protection against disease than raw ones do.

Soul Food Staples in the Phytochemical Medicine Cabinet

Carotenoids and indoles are joined by many other disease-fighting phytochemicals to be found in soul food. Take a look at some of these other phytochemical classes and the foods in which they're found and think about how many of them you use in home cookin'—no matter what part of the country you call home. Allyl sulfides are in onions, garlic, leeks, and chives; saponins are in beans and legumes, such as peanuts and black-eyed peas; phenolic acids are in tomatoes, citrus fruits, carrots, whole grains, and nuts; and terpenes are in cherries and citrus fruit peels.

In days and years to come you'll be hearing more and more about these and other chemical compounds in the phytochemical medicine chest as we learn more about their health benefits. Already there is convincing evidence that they protect us from at least four of the leading causes of death in the United States: diabetes, cardiovascular disease, hypertension, and cancer. In addition to slowing or preventing the reproduction of cancer cells, they help prevent cell damage, decrease cholesterol, and make the blood less likely to clot. That makes for good medicine as well as good eating.

How to Stop Chewing the Fat:
Soul Food Preparation Strategies
to Save Your Life

Meat, Chicken, and More

When I think of soul food in the traditional sense, fat, gravy, and more fat come to mind. If it's meat we want, it must be pan-fried, deep-fried, or smothered in gravy. But half of a fried chicken breast contains about 223 calories and roughly 12 grams of fat. The healthy trick is to cook it in a way that reduces fat and maximizes nutrients. If you oven-fry a breast of the same size, you can reduce the fat content by 6 grams. A 3.5-ounce stewed chicken breast (in a tomato base) can be a low-fat alternative, too, weighing in at just 80 calories and 2.5 grams of fat. Instead of having the requisite high-fat ribs, where a half rack is 492 calories and 40 grams of fat (that's almost the day's total fat allowance for many women), you might opt for a less fatty cut of meat; for instance, a lean loin pork chop has only 170 calories and 7 grams of fat. Better still, although more expensive, is pork tenderloin, a low-fat cut and perhaps the tenderest of all. There are only 200 calories in 3½ ounces of pork tenderloin. What could be better for a big family feast than a pork tenderloin roast accompanied by roasted sweet potatoes, parsnips, and carrots, with a big helping of greens on the side?

Vegetable Soul Food Cookery: Greens

No soul food meal is complete without these leafy vegetables, but we have typically prepared them with ham hocks, fatback, and more salt on top of that. While this creative flavoring may delight your taste buds and bring back fond memories, these high-fat, high-salt foods we've come to crave contribute to hypertension and coronary heart disease, thus negating the benefits of the greens we've added them to. Take my mom, for example. Like many other black women of her generation who'd been reared in the South, she seasoned her greens with ham hocks, fatback, or bacon strips. By doing so, she unknowingly turned a potential nutritional powerhouse into just another food it would be better to avoid. You see, the average serving of greens—whether mustard, collards, or kale—is about 40 to 50 calories when cooked without meat; a 3-ounce serving of watercress is a mere 19 calories; and all greens have negligible amounts of fat. But add 1 ounce of fatback and you add 216 calories to these glorious greens and the fat content goes from nearly 0 to a whopping 23 grams! Try adding what my mom used to call "a strip of lean and a strip of fat," basically fatback with a tiny piece of lean in the middle (it looks like very thick and fatty bacon), and you pile on 216 extra calories and 23.4 grams of fat. Even Stevie Wonder could see the harm in this recipe.

Furthermore, it is well known that in the spirit of giving greens a little soul, we overcook them, simmering for hours and hours until those greens turn brown, rather than the bright to deep green color they are when they still have all the nutrients in them. How many times have you walked into an elderly black woman's home to find a pot of greens simmering in lots of water made greasy with fatback, ham hocks, or neck bones? This practice reduces the greens to a soupy, soggy consistency and leaches the vitamins and minerals right out of them. Unless you drink the pot liquor at the bottom of the pan, where those vitamins and minerals have wound up, you lose almost all the nutritional benefit of the greens.

The more healthful way to prepare greens is to cook them in a small amount of water or fat-free broth only until tender, usually about 20 minutes, so that they retain their healthy vitamins, minerals, and other nutrients rather than losing them to the water. And instead of fatback or ham hocks, we should season our greens with herbs, smoked turkey, onions, garlic, red pepper, and reduced-fat chicken broth. (Check out my "lean greens" recipe in Secret 10—I think you'll find it a great substitute for the traditional greens, and you won't even miss the fat.)

Soul Food Cookery: Cabbage

Cabbage is another soul food vegetable that could help protect us from cancer. Studies in the United States, Japan, and Greece show that people who eat large amounts of cabbage have the lowest rates of colon cancer and tend to have lower death rates overall. We could reap this nutritional benefit, but we lessen our chances when we overcook the cabbage, losing vital vitamin C, a water-soluble vitamin and antioxidant. Even worse, when we cook it in fatback, ham hocks, and bacon grease, we increase the fat content of a great low-fat vegetable, and that, my sista-friend, does not help us in our plight. You've seen cabbage swimming in grease, complete with that requisite piece of fatback or ham hock sitting in the middle of the pot, many a time.

To get the benefits cabbage provides without losing the flavor, replace the fatty meat with low-fat smoked turkey, caraway seeds, and green bell pepper. (See Secret 10 for my recipe.) Alternatively, make a simple coleslaw of shredded red and green cabbage mixed together and bound with a soybean-oil-based mayonnaise or a buttermilk or yogurt dressing.

Soul Food Cookery: Sweet Potatoes

Instead of preparing candied yams, which are loaded with sugar, try making mashed sweet potatoes with orange juice, a sprinkle of brown sugar, skim milk, and reduced-fat butter. Another tasty and healthful option—a sweet potato roasted in its skin with a dash of butter-flavored sprinkles and brown sugar— amounts to only 141 calories and half a gram of fat. But add one pat of butter and 4 tablespoons of sugar and you run up your caloric tab an additional 220 calories. All of a sudden a simple sweet potato, which is so sweet and creamy that it could have been simply baked in its skin without any sugar or fat at all, now costs you a ridiculous 361 calories! See Secret 10 for still another idea about what to do with sweet potatoes. And for a delicious dessert, replace full-fat milk and butter in sweet potato pie with skim milk and butter-flavored extract. You still get great taste, but without the extra fat. The trick with all these foods is to learn how to prepare them so that the extra protection they give us isn't offset by unhealthy ingredients.

Soul Food Cookery: Tomatoes

Since cooked tomatoes, as I mentioned earlier, are more healthful than raw tomatoes, because cooking them releases the cancer-fighting substance lycopene, that old soul food favorite, stewed tomatoes, should stay on your menu. Simply replace butter with reduced-fat butter (which is free of trans fats), and toss in some finely chopped green bell pepper for additional flavor and additional nutrients.

Soul Food Cookery and the Soulful Grain: Corn

I've said throughout this book—and you'll note that I'll keep saying it—that whole grains are good for us. As you read earlier, there is a mountain of evidence to support this claim. But while corn is a grain and we do like our corn bread, we have got to start to make it and eat it with less fat. We can also increase the nutritional and lifesaving potential of this soul food by increasing its fiber content. Simply add whole-kernel corn to your bread. And that's not all: Throw in a handful of chopped red and green bell peppers and maybe a dash of minced jalapeño peppers for extra zest. The point is to add some vegetables and some color so that you get more fiber, more disease-fighting antioxidants, and more phytochemicals—and a bigger flavor hit, too.

Soul Food Cookery: Holiday Chitlins

A word about choices. When it comes to holidays like Christmas, Thanksgiving, and New Year's, I know there are a great number of black folks who like their chitlins. While I truly believe there are no good or bad foods, these pig intestines contain a colossal serving of fat. At 1,105 calories and 59.11 grams of fat per 8-ounce serving (and most folks typically eat more than 8 ounces in one sitting), this is not a good food choice. Have it at your own risk. And please, don't do it more than once a year. Even then, ease up on the portion size. A better idea might be to have a thin slice of Grandma's homemade sweet potato pie instead. Check the chart below of "old soul foods" choices versus "new soul foods" choices for other healthy food switches you can make.

Table 4-1 Traditional Soul Foods and Their New Counterparts

Old Soul Foods	New Soul Foods
Candied sweet potatos (361 cal; 12 g fat)	Baked sweet potato in skin (141 cal; 1 g fat)
Greens with fatback, ham hocks (256 cal; 23 g fat)	Greens seasoned with vegetable broth and herbs (65 cal; 1 g fat

Old Soul Foods	New Soul Foods
Macaroni and (full-fat) cheese with eggs (453 cal; 11 g fat)	Mac and cheese with low-fat cheese, egg whites, and bread crumbs (194 cal; 2 g fat)
Southern fried chicken breast (223 cal; 12 g fat)	Oven-fried chicken (201 cal; 6 g fat)
Cabbage with ham hocks (186 cal; 14 g fat)	Cabbage with fresh dill (60 cal; 0 g fat)
White rice and gravy (246 cal; 7.2 g fat)	Brown rice and black beans (268 cal; 1.4 g fat)
Fried apples (270 cal; 12 g fat)	Steamed apples and cinnamon (150 cal; 1 g fat)
Fried potatoes and onions (230 cal; 12 g fat)	Steamed potatoes and onions with red and green bell peppers (92 cal; 3.6 g fat)
Butter beans with ham hocks (407 cal; 19 g fat)	Lima beans with stevia and reduced-fat butter (111 cal; 1 g fat)
Smothered pork chops (396 cal; 29.5 g fat)	Caribbean-style pork tenderloin (200 calories; 4 g fat)

Frequently Asked Questions

Q Dr. Ro: You say we shouldn't use fatback and pork fat to season our vegetables, but I'm confused over which kind of fat or oil I should use. So many of the dishes my mom and grandmother taught me to cook make use of those fats. What should I replace them with?

A *Monounsaturated fats such as olive, canola, and peanut oil and polyunsaturated fats such as corn, safflower, and soybean oils are all believed to reduce your risk of heart disease because they lower LDL (bad) cholesterol and raise HDL (good) cholesterol. More recently the scientific community has also touted the health benefits of adding grape-seed oil and flaxseed oil to your diet. You might like to know that flaxseed oil aids in protecting your skin against the aging process, but it may have more general anti-aging effects, too, because it is particularly high in omega-3 fatty acids, which have benefits for cells and for cell processes throughout your body. Some studies suggest that omega-3 fatty acids help to prevent blood platelets from clotting and sticking to artery walls, reducing the risk of heart attacks and strokes. Walnut oil, soybean oil, and canola oil are also relatively high in omega-3s. So take your choice from among olive, canola, peanut, corn, safflower, soybean, flaxseed, walnut, and grape-seed oils. Some have quite distinct tastes, while others are almost completely neutral. Corn and safflower oils are better for frying. Experiment and see which you like.*

While I encourage you to use any of the oils listed

*above, you should try to cut back on cooking with satu-
rated fats, which are found in animal products such as
lard, butter, bacon grease, and fatback (and in a few
vegetable oils like palm and coconut oil), because saturated fats raise LDL levels in your body, thus reversing
the benefits of a healthful diet. However, at the same
time that they raise LDL levels, saturated fats also raise
HDL levels. In this respect they are at least better than
the trans fats, which are found in shortening, in stick
margarines, and in anything that lists partially hydrogenated oil among its ingredients, because the trans fats
raise only the bad LDL cholesterol and have been found
to have a significant impact on heart disease. So if you
like to cook or season foods with margarine, be sure to
read the label carefully to make certain it is one of the
brands that is free of trans fats and high in polyunsaturated fat.*

*Another thing to think of as you're cooking those veg-
etables: Why not try expanding your horizons in the
kitchen by also seasoning with herbs, spices, juices from
fruits and vegetables, and fat-free broths? This way you
can drastically reduce or eliminate the amount of fat you
need to add to create a flavorful dish. For example, dill
is wonderful with cabbage. It enhances the flavor, and
frankly, you won't miss the meat. If you fancy smoke-
flavored foods, sometimes you might add just a hint of
liquid smoke, but be careful, as it really masks the flavor
of produce. Adding sun-dried tomatoes, or lemon or orange juice is also a great way to wake up the flavor in
foods. Apple juice, raisins, and a little brown sugar or ste-
via (a natural calorie-free sweetener) work wonders on
sweet potatoes if you're longing for candied sweets. Be*

creative with your choices, and don't be afraid to try new combinations that you never thought would work. Often they do!

Q   Dr. Ro: I am from Louisiana, where we cook with a lot of peppers and garlic. My family uses both. Can I tell them that these foods help our health? How?

A   *Garlic is a vegetable in the genus* Allium, *which contains roughly 25 or so chemical compounds that fight viruses, bacteria, and fungi. Some experts recommend eating at least one raw clove of garlic a day—or several cloves, if you feel a cold coming on. Like tomatoes and watermelon, red bell peppers contain a chemical compound called lycopene, which protects against cancer. I know that in your region hot peppers are popular, too. While I'm not aware of any particular nutritional benefit, they do contain a substance called capsaicin, which is used in many topical pain medications.*

Secret 5

The Truth About the Most Popular Diet and Weight Loss Plans

We live in a myth-loving society when it comes to weight loss and other matters of our health. And it doesn't help that even the scientists are always changing their minds. There's not a day that goes by that doesn't bring about a new set of commandments about healthy eating. If you try to keep up with the latest expert advice, as I do, your head will spin from all the contradictions. One day margarine is good; the next day it's a hydrogenated fat and way bad. One day alcohol is dangerous; the next we're almost ordered to drink a glass of wine with dinner—and that dinner had better be carbohydrate-free, even though a few years ago we were told to eat pasta and forget meat.

Okay, I'm exaggerating, but you get the point. There are so many myths and pieces of misinformation floating around that it's no wonder you're asking: Can I eat potatoes and still lose weight? Could a spoonful of apple cider vinegar really help me drop pounds? Can I really eat as much fat as I want? And, like the Energizer Bunny, the questions just keep comin' and comin'—because changes in the answers we get from the experts just keep comin', too. Well, rest easy. You won't have to buy another diet book, because the common-sense information you'll find in this chapter will help you evaluate for yourself how to separate the wheat from the chaff—the whole wheat, that is! The truth about what works may need some fine-tuning over the years, but there's a lot of us in the field of nutrition who are in basic agreement about what doesn't work—the myths that govern much of our eating and dietary behavior.

Six of these myths about diets and foods involve "miracle" weight loss diets shared at the office water cooler, on the Internet, over the phone lines, and in many best-selling diet books. Your girlfriends swear by them, but by the next week they always seem to be on to yet another new diet, " 'cause, girl, this one just ain't working anymore"—which is why I call them dud diets. The other five myths consist of various beliefs about food-based shortcuts to health or weight loss that are either oversimplifications or out-and-out falsehoods—which is why I call them food fallacies.

The dud diets and food fallacies are many and long-lasting—so much so that I could probably do an entire book just on them alone. But I've chosen seven of the most popular diet plans and five of the most prevalent weight loss myths to illustrate my point about how we allow ourselves to be misled in our desperate quest for quick fixes. Here are my six top picks for dud diets.

Dud Diets

Dud Diet #1: Grapefruit Diet

If you like fruit, this one is a doozy. But despite their tartness (and in spite of what you've heard from your best friend's aunt), grapefruits don't "dry up" or "suck out" body fat.

How the Diet Works: ✦ The Grapefruit Diet comes in many varieties. Basically, you eat half a grapefruit before each meal, and your calories are generally limited to fewer than 800 a day, although some versions of the diet do encourage you to eat until you're full. The diet, which usually lasts for one to three weeks, does not allow alcohol but encourages caffeine intake. The rationale for the diet? Supposedly you benefit from the grapefruit's fat-burning enzymes. But the quick weight loss that this diet promotes, like that of many fad diets, is due mostly to the loss of water—and, of course, to the 800 calories or fewer that you are eating. The reason caffeine is encouraged is because it, too, promotes water loss. Caffeine is like a diuretic (a fluid pill), which sends you to the bathroom, flushing your system of water. But if you want to lose anything besides water, this is not the diet for you.

What Makes the Diet a Dud: ✦ The Grapefruit Diet is a low-calorie diet that is also low in protein, fiber, and important vitamins and minerals. If you remember nothing more about the diet games people play, please know this: Diets that encourage you to focus on a single food will always give you short shrift. Why?

Because there really is no perfect food, no one food item that can provide all of the nutrients your body needs, in the correct amounts you need, to be healthy. So when a diet promotes a single food as its base, it will always, by its very nature, fall short of its promise. It is true that grapefruit is a rich source of vitamin C, and pink and red grapefruit are good sources of beta-carotene, which protects against cancer. And it's also true that grapefruits, as a part of a wholesome and varied diet, are a good food to eat regularly. But they certainly aren't a strong enough foundation for a healthy diet. Nor can an 800-calorie grapefruit-based diet help you to achieve long-term weight loss. As soon as the diet is over, you will go back to eating the foods you used to eat, and the weight loss is, well, lost. And for the record, there is no scientific proof that grapefruit actually contains fat-burning enzymes. So my advice is to include it in your list of healthful fruits and vegetables, make it a part of your whole dietary picture, and move on to real success.

Dud Diet #2: Cabbage Soup Diet

Now, don't get me wrong, I like cabbage as much as the next girl, but soup made of cabbage, consumed as the mainstay of your diet, amounts to sheer boredom in my book. And, like the grapefruit diet, it's nonsense because, although it does allow a few other foods, it's still a mainly one-food diet.

How the Diet Works: ✦ The Cabbage Soup Diet allows you to eat as much cabbage as you want for about 7 to 10 days. The claim is that you'll lose up to 15 pounds. Although there are variations of this diet, there is a basic recipe for making the soup, its main component. Essentially, you mix a variety of low-calorie vegetables, like cabbage, onions, and tomatoes (sometimes carrots), and flavor the mix with bouillon, onion soup mix, and tomato juice. Every day of the seven-day program, in addition to the cabbage soup, you have to eat very specific foods, such as potatoes, fruit juice, and vegetables; on one day, you're allowed to eat 10 to 20 ounces of beef. Yes, you lose weight, and you lose it quickly. And why wouldn't you? First, consider that your calorie count is way down after eating mainly low-cal soup. Then consider that most of your weight loss is due to—you guessed it—water. And you pay a sometimes hefty price for this water loss.

What Makes the Diet a Dud: ✦ The Cabbage Soup Diet is too low in complex carbohydrates and protein, not to mention vitamins and minerals. For this reason it cannot be maintained for any extended period of time. It causes light-headedness, weakness, and a reduced ability to concentrate. Imagine trying to stay on this diet when you're studying for a major exam or preparing for an intense challenge at work. Good luck! Weakness and disorientation are just the main reported side effects of this diet. Try adding nausea and heavy gas to the mix as well. Doesn't sound like fun anymore, does it?

Dud Diet #3: Eating for Your Blood Type

Okay, folks, this seems interesting at first glance. And I admit, it is different from traditional wisdom. In fact, it defies wisdom—and logic. Puh-leeze! While a family may have varying blood types within its ranks, do you honestly believe you can be so different in your nutritional requirements that each of you has to shop for, cook, and eat different foods? How absurd! (Not to mention time-consuming and expensive.)

How the Diet Works: ✦ Of the four basic blood types known, each has a different list of food groups that must be avoided. Eliminating entire food groups is often recommended on the grounds that these foods will cause weight gain or simply be bad for you. Red flag, people! When you are cautioned against an entire food group, ask yourself whether or not the "expert" is really giving you helpful advice. The reason? Foods are organized into groups by virtue of the various nutrients they contain. You need the nutrients in all of these groups working together as a team to achieve optimal health. No single food group should be banned from a diet. To the contrary, we need all of them for normal body functions, like growing hair and nails, repairing skin, strengthening bones, and helping us see better. If you eliminate an entire food group, you weaken the team, making it hard for the remaining team members to do their jobs for you.

Eating for your blood type presumes that your blood type has a unique antigen marker that reacts negatively to certain foods. According to this diet, people with varying digestive systems and enzymes and different stomach acid levels must be correlated with specific blood types. If only nature were that simple. Believe me, it's not.

What Makes the Diet a Dud: ✦ For starters, before we even get to the health issues, the Blood Type Diet is grossly inconsiderate of a family's pocketbook. If each member must eat different foods according to his or her blood type, we'd all go broke on the grocery bill alone. And how confusing would it be to try to eat a meal out or plan a party according to this diet? The main point is that there are no studies to support the premise that diet should be based on a person's blood type. Further, the diet is hugely restrictive because you must follow a list of foods you can and cannot eat. I don't know about you, but being bossed around to this degree would make me want to eat more of everything! And again, when you specifically limit or restrict groups of foods, as this diet dictates, you set yourself up for nutrient deficiency. One more thing: When's the last time you checked your blood type? You don't know what it is, do you? That's just as I thought. Not to worry. Most of the weight loss with this plan is found in the pile of foods you can't eat. Bottom line? You eat so few foods that you can't help but shed a few pounds. The question is, can you keep them off? Will they come back when you go back to eating your favorites again? The answer is yes to both questions.

Dud Diet #4: Food Combining

There is one good thing about this diet: It encourages you to eat copious amounts of fruits and vegetables. And you probably will lose weight because of that factor alone. Remember, fruits and vegetables are among the lowest-calorie foods available to us. But there's just one problem . . . well, maybe a couple.

How the Diet Works: ✦ The Food Combining Diet requires that roughly 70 percent of the foods you eat be fruits and vegetables. The remaining 30 percent of the foods should consist of one or two servings of starch, in the form of rice or pasta, with minimal animal protein. You can't consume dairy products at all. And the diet discourages the use of alcohol and caffeine (a good thing). Those who recommend this diet claim that you lose weight when you eat the foods in the proper combinations, when in actuality, if you lose weight on this diet, you can be sure it's because you're eating mostly low-calorie foods—fruits and veggies.

What Makes the Diet a Dud: ✦ The Food Combining Diet is deficient in important nutrients: protein, calcium, zinc, and vitamins D and B_{12}. Again, here's the all-too-familiar concept of cutting out a food group. This time it's dairy. And meat, chicken, and fish are practically eliminated, too. Hence the calcium and protein shortcomings of this diet. Now, *real* food combining, which is supported by science but is completely different from what is known as the Food Combining Diet, recommends that you combine foods in the same meal to maximize their potential to be used by the body. Take, for example, eating oranges with steak or having a glass of orange juice with a serving of collard greens. The idea is that the vitamin C in the fruit or juice increases the body's ability to make use of the iron in the steak and the greens. In other words, the body better absorbs iron-rich foods when you eat them in the same meal with a serving of a food rich in vitamin C. But with the fad version of this diet, you're not combining foods that have been scientifically proven to complement each other; you're simply eliminating certain foods—as well as nutrients.

Dud Diet #5: High-Protein, Low-Carb Diets

High-protein, low-carb plans such as the Atkins Diet have been very popular, with many people swearing that they lost weight. But if these diets really work, why are Americans fatter than we've ever been? At a time when two-thirds of the country is overweight, many obese (and when black women are overweight at the alarmingly high rate of 50 percent), we have to ask ourselves what's really going on here. I've combed the barrage of information and data available, and I've personally talked to hundreds of people who've tried these diets. For some they actually worked.

Well, sort of. They worked for a time. But you have to hear, as I have, the numerous stories of eventual disappointment, the stories sistas tell when they've "tried all they could try, done all they could do," only to lose and then regain those same 10, 20, or 50 pounds. Again.

Here's my take on the high-protein smoke-and-mirrors diets.

How the Diet Works: ✦ The High-Protein Diets operate on the basic premise that you can lose weight by consuming between 30 to 40 percent of your daily calories each from protein and fat, and the rest from carbohydrates. On most versions of this diet, high-carb foods such as sugars, pasta, bread, potatoes, and cereals are a no-no or have to be kept to an absolute minimum, while red meat and other animal proteins, as well as cheese, eggs, and as much fat as you like, are encouraged. There are many variations of the High-Protein Diet, but suffice it to say that most work on the assumption that when you eat foods containing high amounts of carbohydrates in either starch or sugar form, your body responds by making too much insulin too fast, and the insulin causes you to store excess calories as fat. But when it comes to excess carbs leading to weight gain, the fact is that a calorie is a calorie is a calorie, whether those calories are from carbohydrates, proteins, or fats. So my feeling is that one of the basic premises for this diet as a route to weight loss is flawed. And while we're on the subject of the anti-carb biases of these high-protein diets, it should be pointed out that most of them do not distinguish between refined and whole-grain carbs. As discussed in Secret 3, whole-grain carbohydrates are much superior to refined and don't cause the rise in insulin and blood sugar that the protein folks hold up as their rationale for their anti-carb stance. Instead of beating up on carbs, they should be concerned about the high level of saturated fats contained in the animal foods they recommend in these diets, which are a far more serious health threat than carbs—putting you at risk for heart disease, high blood pressure, diabetes, and more.

Perhaps the biggest problem with most of these high-protein diets is that it is next to impossible to stay on them for the long term, which is precisely what you'd have to do in order to keep the pounds off.

Breaking Down High-Protein Diets

Atkins ✦ If you've joined the ranks of those looking for a "diet revolution," you might even have lost a lot of weight on one or another version of this diet. With Atkins, for example, you tend to consume fewer calories, even though the diet is high in fat, because the high-fat foods the diet encourages stave off hunger longer than lower-fat foods. This means you'll be less inclined to raid the fridge than a person who eats more-healthful foods. Remember, as I've said many times, the key to weight loss is consuming fewer calories.

But a major drawback of this diet is that it contains far fewer fruits, vegetables, legumes, and whole grains than it should. It is, therefore, lower in vital nutrients such as calcium, antioxidants, and fiber, all of which keep chronic disease at bay. Again, not only is eating more fruits and vegetables a healthful practice, but in the long run it will contribute to weight loss. Think about it. Most fruits and a number of colorful vegetables have a higher water content than do calorically dense, high-fat foods. The more water a food contains, the fewer calories it contains. Translation? By eating fruits and vegetables, you can eat greater quantities of food while still losing weight, and also give your health a big boost through all the vitamins, nutrients, and fiber you'll be taking in.

What Makes the Diet a Dud: ✦ In the beginning weeks of the Atkins diet, the weight loss is mostly due to fluids. Later, weight loss includes fat, and finally, if you stay on the diet long enough, muscle. On the Atkins diet there are very few carbohydrates to choose from—initially only 20 grams a day, about 230 grams less than most people typically consume—so your body quickly resorts to its fat stores for energy, which, of course, results in weight loss. But eventually it may also dip into its protein stores—in other words, it may rob from your muscles, resulting in a condition called muscle wasting, which can have dangerous effects on your health. Some of the adverse health effects of muscle wasting include heart malfunctions such as irregular heartbeat.

Because of the high-protein, low-carbohydrate content of the diet, you may also be at risk for kidney damage. Then there's the calcium issue, too. High-protein diets leach calcium out of the bones—and African Americans already don't get enough calcium in our diets. As noted above, the high saturated fat and cholesterol content of the diet is also a virtual blueprint for heart disease, clogging arteries and leading to heart attacks and strokes, which is why the American Heart Association is among its many critics. At a time when African Americans suffer alarmingly high rates of these diseases, this is a risk, my sistas, we cannot afford to take.

Now, if you are thinking, "My girlfriend went on this diet and she lost a lot of weight and nothing happened to her," I must ask you how long she remained on the diet and how long she kept the weight off. This, like so many other diets, cannot sustain long-term weight loss because people just don't stay on it for long.

In a survey that followed 80,000 people back in 1982 and again 10 years later, the people who were most likely to gain weight were frequent meat eaters, those who ate meat seven times or more each week. Those people who followed a vegetable-rich diet containing 19 or more servings a week and who walked or ran up to four hours a week were most likely to lose weight. According to this and other evidence, the combination of vegetables and exercise is a powerful force for weight loss and for good health overall.

Even if by chance you do know people who have lost weight on the Atkins diet and kept it off, the long-term health effects of this kind of eating have not been studied enough to prove that it is not harmful to us. Until that proof is offered, I will continue to recommend that you eat more (not fewer) fruits, vegetables, legumes, and whole grains, and move your body for successful and long-term weight loss and maintenance. As a scientist, I must tell you that Dr. Atkins may have said his diet works, but in God I trust. All others must have data!

The Zone ✦ In the zone. Sounds like a cool place to be, doesn't it? The zone is actually the place where insulin levels are supposed to stay within an "acceptable range" based on a caloric distribution of 40-30-30— that is, 40 percent of your calories coming from carbohydrates, 30 percent from protein, and 30 percent from fat. The protein foods included in the diet are mostly low-fat foods, like cottage cheese, fish, and chicken breast. On this diet, less than 10 percent of your fat calories should come from saturated (the bad artery-clogging) fat. The plan is supposed to give the dieter energy.

What Makes the Diet a Dud: ✦ This diet does cause weight loss because on it you consume very few calories—generally 1,000 a day, though it can range up to 1,600 daily. But the diet has a lot of problems. It is short on complex carbohydrates, which provide real energy. It is low in fiber (a common fault of nearly all these diets) and low in vitamins and minerals, primarily because pasta, potatoes, and whole-grain breads and cereals are also restricted. Further, it is low in calcium, a mineral also typically found in lower than the recommended amounts in the diets of black folks. Another drawback: If you don't like counting numbers and keeping track of the value of everything you eat, this diet can be difficult to follow. If you like eating bagels by the quarter portion, 2 ounces of cheese at a time, or half an apple, the Zone might be the diet for you. If you like to eat foods you enjoy without a strict meal plan, then skip it altogether.

Dud Diet #6: Sugar Busters

This diet says that refined (white) sugar, the kind found in cakes, pies, other desserts, and soda, and refined carbohydrates, the kind found in white bread and in processed grains such as white rice, are toxic and cause automatic weight gain. Supposedly the extra pounds are due to increased amounts of insulin, which the diet's creators say produces increased amounts of body fat. For the record, sugar provides empty calories, so there is no real nutritional benefit, but to call it toxic stretches the truth. Even the American Diabetes Association says that no carbohydrate has to be forbidden entirely, even for diabetics.

According to the association, what matters most in terms of causing insulin and blood sugar to spike is the total amount of carbs, not their type or food source. Bottom line? I think Sugar Busters is on to a good thing in its effort to get people to eat less sugar and fewer refined foods. But the Sugar Busters Diet is not a perfect plan for reasons I'll describe below. Still, it's a much better bet than some of the high-protein diet varieties, which could actually be dangerous to your health, and which are extremely unlikely to result in long-term weight loss.

How the Diet Works ✦ On the Sugar Busters Diet, you eat foods with a low glycemic index—which means foods that are digested slowly and therefore don't cause sudden, rapid spikes in blood sugar and insulin. That's the point of eating whole grains and dried beans, as well as green vegetables and certain fruits, like cantaloupe, blueberries, apples, oranges, and grapefruit. You must avoid foods considered to have a high glycemic index—carrots, corn, beets, potatoes (except sweet potatoes), rice, white bread, pasta, bananas, watermelon, raisins, a few other fruits, and all foods that contain refined sugar—cakes, pies, candy, soda, and other sweets.

What Makes the Diet a Dud: ✦ Yes, most people in America consume about a pound of sugar a week. That's certainly more than we need, and far more empty calories than are necessary to achieve optimal health. But there is absolutely no scientific evidence to support the theory that refined sugar, consumed in modest quantities, makes for automatic weight gain in all people. Further, this business of eliminating potatoes, pasta, bananas, and other specific fruits from the diet so they become part of a "forbidden foods" list is just plain bunk! Don't blame the pasta and the potatoes; it's the butter, sour cream, and cheese-laden cream sauces we load on top of these two much-maligned foods that are the real culprits here.

This diet is built, in theory, on a good idea—reducing consumption of sugar and refined starches. But to advise eliminating healthful foods such as bananas, watermelon, carrots, corn, potatoes, and pasta is misleading. Even more crucial, and the problem that makes the diet unlikely to result in weight loss for most people, is that there is not much direction given for controlling portion size beyond a couple of admonitions to be "moderate." Obviously, if you don't pay attention to portions, it's an easy plan to follow, but a hard one to lose weight on.

Popular Food Fallacies: Everything You Need to Know to Debunk Them

I know you've heard of them. You've probably even believed a few of them yourself. You know what I'm talking about: the "wisdom" of old women in the family, your girlfriends, sistas at the office, or nosy neighbors. I call these my top five picks among the many pieces of misinformation that we sistas have swallowed hook, line, and sinker all in the name of weight loss and good health.

Food Fallacy #1: Milk Makes Black People Big Fat Cows

One of my personal favorites in the world of food fallacies (which are usually seeded with a grain of truth) is the hype surrounding the potential for dairy products to destroy the health of the black family, as though there were some conspiracy underfoot.

There seems to be a misunderstanding floating through much of the black community. Somehow, the theory that black bodies were not made to digest milk has gained widespread acceptance, creating a mountain of confusion, not to mention ill-founded paranoia. The idea that getting black folks to drink milk is some sort of conspiracy by the government and by farmers to kill us off prematurely is, of course, preposterous. Still, many black people believe this to be true. I have personally heard the theory aired ad nauseum on talk radio and during panel discussions at sista-circle weekends; even some of my viewers have broached the subject with me. This would not be an issue except that it has become yet another contributor to uninformed health practices on our part and, as a result, sets us up for nutritional deficiency.

Is milk bad for black people? No. But there is some truth to the notion that milk may cause discomfort for some of us.

Truth Grain

It is a fact that about 75 percent of African Americans in the United States may not produce an enzyme called lactase. If a person doesn't have lactase, this can lead to a condition called lactose intolerance.

Since lactose is the sugar contained in milk, a person who doesn't produce lactase will not be able to properly digest milk. Being lactose-intolerant can cause cramps, gas, bloating, and diarrhea.

Though many people produce enough lactase in the proper quantities throughout life and don't have any digestive problems with milk, other people produce the enzyme only during infancy and early childhood years. As they grow older they usually stop drinking as much milk as they did at a younger age.

If you consistently experience feelings of discomfort such as those mentioned above after drinking milk or consuming other dairy products, you should consult a doctor. Refrain from diagnosing yourself, because the symptoms of lactose intolerance could also be due to some other health problem. Lactose intolerance can be diagnosed by a medical test that measures blood sugar levels after a dose of lactose is taken by mouth. If your plasma glucose level increases by less than 20 mg/dl, then you probably are lactose intolerant.

If it turns out that you are, that does not mean that you should stop drinking milk or eating dairy products. Black folks' diets already lack sufficient calcium and other important minerals; we can ill afford to cut out a whole food group that provides an excellent source of vital nutrients. Still, when three-fourths of the African American population has problems digesting dairy products, the problem must be addressed.

There are a number of things you can do to get around the problem. First, you need to know that there are products on the market for you, such as lactose-free and lactose-reduced milk. These provide the same amount of calcium and other nutrients found in their traditional counterparts. You may also opt to take Lactaid (which you can buy over the counter in any drug or grocery story) as a supplement just before eating or drinking dairy products. Finally, if you are still leery of dairy products, you can get calcium from canned sardines and canned salmon eaten with the bones. And you will see, as you read upcoming chapters, that I have also found other ways of dealing with the problem in my Livin' Healthy Plan, which includes not only lots of vegetables but other foods that are good sources of calcium. Calcium-enriched soy products such as tofu, which are one of the basics of my eating plan, are particularly terrific sources of calcium for those of us who don't like milk or don't digest it well.

Like it or not, calcium is a bigger concern than you might think. In fact, since we suffer hypertension disproportionately, we are in particular need of calcium, because it's now known to be an important factor in controlling blood pressure. A growing number of studies tell us that when calcium is low in the diet, blood pressure is high, and when calcium is increased, blood pressure goes down. This has been demonstrated over and over again in animal studies, and calcium's effect on blood pressure seems to be borne out by human studies as well. Researchers looked at the blood pressures and calcium consumption of over 1,700 black and white women and men. They found a general trend toward lower blood pressure levels in those people who consumed more milk and yogurt, both high-calcium foods. A diet rich in calcium seems to counteract the adverse effects of a high-sodium diet, which is thought to be related to hypertension. But to protect yourself even better from high blood pressure, your diet should be both calcium-rich and low in sodium.

Getting an adequate amount of calcium in the diet is particularly important for pregnant women, because it is very likely that calcium can provide protection against hypertension not only throughout adulthood but for future generations. Animal studies indicate that when high-calcium diets are consumed during pregnancy and during breast-feeding, the baby is protected from high blood pressure. But the opposite is true when expectant mothers consume low-calcium diets.

Food Fallacy #2: Lemon Juice and Vinegar Suck Up Body Fat and Lower Blood Pressure

Another of my favorite myths is the idea that lemon juice and vinegar somehow suck out or dry up fat. Here's a true story. I was speaking at a university, and before going to the stage to deliver my keynote speech, I was greeted by a small group of sistas who gathered outside the auditorium. One of them approached, asking if I was Dr. Ro of *Heart and Soul*, and when I said I was, she gently pulled me aside to share a "secret."

"I know you answer a lot of questions on your show. You've helped me many times, so I thought I'd return the favor," she whispered.

"Well, spill it, girl," I replied, eager to know what she had to say.

"Look," she said, "my girlfriend got her blood pressure down with lemon juice, vinegar, and garlic. It worked because the lemon juice and vinegar helped her to lose the weight."

"How'd it do that?" I asked.

"You see, it melted the pounds away, and her blood pressure went down. Now she's all better! Isn't that marvelous?" she exclaimed, waiting for my sanction. "Now you can use this on your show. Don't forget to tell them to use fresh garlic and lemons."

To get my sista-friend to understand that lemons and vinegar neither suck out nor dry up fat was an exercise in futility. She was convinced, because she believed it had worked for her girlfriend. But here's my word on vinegar and lemon juice: The fact that a food is tart does not mean it is conducive to fat or weight loss. And if you have high blood pressure, it's not a remedy for that, either. The body doesn't work that way.

Truth Grain: ✦ Lemons do contain a mineral, potassium, that has the ability to lower blood pressure. But don't stop taking your blood pressure medicine because your friend thinks lemon juice is the answer. That is not a safe health practice. The same goes for garlic, which may also lower blood pressure as well as reduce your cholesterol. Scientists believe certain substances in garlic relax smooth muscles in the artery walls, allowing blood to flow through arteries unhampered. One study found that garlic lowered the diastolic blood pressure of mildly hypertensive men by an average of 11 points. So my advice is to eat lemon and garlic as preventive measures—and maybe you'll never have to take blood pressure medication. But if your doctor has put you on one of those drugs, don't think lemon and garlic can do the job by themselves. And don't expect to lose weight by just adding lemon or garlic to your diet, either. They're not magical substances.

Food Fallacy #3: Drinking Juice Is an Effective Weight Loss Strategy

Since we're on the subject of juice, allow me to deal with another popular myth. Some of us think juice is the answer to peeling off pounds. How many times have you heard that if you'd just put down the fork and put your blender to work, you could be in weight loss heaven? I have heard this theory many times. In fact, it is so popular that it should be explained here, once and for all, that even juice has calories.

Truth Grain: ✦ It is true that fruit and vegetable juices contain vitamins and antioxidants (disease-fighting chemicals) that are good for you. But a well-rounded diet is not one-dimensional. It contains foods from a variety of sources, which are found in more than one food group. Even within the same food group some choices are better than others. And in the case of juices, they are not as good for you as the foods they come from. This is because ounce for nutritious ounce, juice provides more calories than its whole fruit and vegetable counterparts, and without the fiber.

A 16-ounce glass of cranberry juice will cost you about 300 calories, give you no fiber, and offer only a slim chance of staving off hunger. So in the long run it will do little to keep unwanted pounds at bay. Compare a 6-ounce serving of apple juice to a medium apple with its skin. While the apple juice provides 90 calories and a paltry 0.2 grams of fiber, the medium apple, by contrast, contains only 81 calories but gives you 3.7 grams of fiber, including soluble fiber, which provides an added benefit by protecting you against heart disease. The fiber also gives you a feeling of fullness, so you don't get hungry five minutes later and head straight to the fridge for a raid. A juice diet, on the other hand, will leave you hungry and provide your body with less much-needed nutrients contained in greater amounts in the whole foods from which the juice originates in the first place.

Food Fallacy #4: Fasting Helps Peel Off Pounds

According to noted nutritional anthropologist Dr. Shiriki Kumanyika, black women tend to believe it is safe and acceptable to fast or starve ourselves as a weight loss strategy. Because of our cultural and religious beliefs, fasting fits what we do as a community. It appeals to the scores of sistas who long for a holistic health practice that will address our problems.

Truth Grain: ✦ The trouble with fasting as a way to lose weight is that it amounts to little more than starving yourself into fatness. Why? Because when you starve yourself, you are in effect telling your body to get ready for the famine, which causes it to hold on to whatever calories you do give it much more tenaciously than it usually does. This happens because the Creator has made your body a very efficient organism.

Remember what I told you about the thrifty gene: To protect you from those times when food is in short supply, the body goes into survival mode. Simply put, if there is insufficient food for sustenance, your body will protect itself by lowering your basal metabolic rate—the number of calories your body needs to maintain itself at rest—so that it takes fewer calories to survive. Eating very low-calorie diets or nothing at all can reduce your BMR by as much as 35 percent, and that lower metabolic rate may persist long after the diet is over, making it much harder to lose weight over the long term. There are other downsides to this practice, too.

When your body moves into survival mode, you run the risk of losing lean muscle. Once it has used up its ready supply of fat stores, the body breaks your muscle tissue down to use for fuel to meet energy needs. You need this fuel to take the kids to school and to go to work or school yourself, to say nothing of normal body functions like breathing, walking, talking, sweating, and just moving around doing what you must to live. Because muscle tissue burns calories much more efficiently than fat, the result of this muscle wasting is that you are not able to burn calories as well as you did before you started your starvation routine. And with your body burning calories more slowly than before, you're headed for piling *on* pounds, not shaving them off.

Starving yourself has yet another drawback. When you eat so few calories, you set yourself up for nutrient deficiency. Sure, experts often recommend liquid meals-in-a-can, but they are useful only as supplements to a healthful diet, not as meal replacements. In the long run the only thing you can count on through fasting is that nutrient deficiencies over time will damage your body and calorie deficiencies will slow down your body's ability to burn calories in the future. The result is that you'll gain weight. So what am I saying here? In order to lose weight, you've got to get your eat on!

You must first eat enough food (and preferably the good-for-you variety) to be healthy. With weight loss as your goal, you can safely reduce your daily caloric level to 500 calories less than your average daily requirement needs, which will help you to lose weight at a safe rate of one pound each week. So if you require 2,000 calories for normal body maintenance, to lose a pound a week you'll need to cut back to 1,500 calories a day. Take a look at Secret 2 for a review of how to calculate your BMR and your daily caloric needs.

Don't despair and throw in the towel at the thought of losing "only" a pound a week. Remember, this is about living for the long term. In case I need to remind you, the pyramids weren't built in a day; neither were those thighs. So let's concentrate on losing for health and keeping the weight off in an effort to be fit, not fat.

Food Fallacy #5: Pasta, Bread, Potatoes, and Other Carbohydrates Make You Fat

You've heard the expression "don't hate the player, hate the game"? It's appropriate in this case. Bread, pasta, and potatoes are not the enemies. It's the butter, cream, and other high-fat toppings we heap on these nutrient-packed, energizing foods that do us in.

Potatoes are a nutrient- and fiber-rich food that fills you up quickly and, ounce for ounce, has far fewer calories than the sugar-laden foods we consume in such large amounts. Sweet potatoes are especially nutritious and good for you—if eaten without marshmallows! Cooked correctly and consumed in moderation, potatoes, breads, and pastas (particularly if the breads and pastas are made with whole grains) are nutrient- and carbohydrate-dense foods that provide a good source of energy as well as B vitamins and iron. They make you feel fuller faster, so you are less likely to overeat than if you're eating ice cream, cookies, or cake.

Truth Grain: ✦ You may have heard that carbohydrates are not body-friendly, because when your body has its fill of carbs, it turns the leftovers into fat. Here's a news flash: All foods are eventually converted to blood sugar and ultimately stored as fat if the calories you consume exceed the calories you burn.

When it comes to eating carbohydrates while you're trying to lose weight, I say eat up! Just make sure that you're eating whole-grain carbs, in the form of whole wheat, barley, bulgur, brown rice, oats, quinoa (pronounced "keen-wa"), couscous (a Mediterranean grain that looks a little like yellow grits and has a slightly grainier texture), and buckwheat.

Go back to your grandmother's favorite recipes and make your pancakes using whole-wheat or buckwheat flour, then add oats to them. Think or eat outside the box and try new favorites, like one of my favorites, tabouli, a Mediterranean salad made with bulgur and other healthful goodies such as tomatoes, olive oil, green onions, and mint. Have brown rice with your black beans. Add whole-grain carbs to soups, salads, meatloaf, and other mixed dishes. To lose weight, the trick is to eat foods that are bulky relative to their calorie content and so provide a feeling of fullness for a relatively small caloric cost. They're also packed with nutrients. And if you add large amounts of fresh fruits and vegetables to them to complete your meal, you get an even bigger bang for your caloric as well as nutritional buck. In the end you've eaten a lot of nutritious food, you're full, and you've consumed fewer calories than you would have had you opted for high-fat foods, which on average are more than twice as calorie-dense, ounce for ounce, as carbohydrates.

Is There Such a Thing as a Successful Diet?

In a chapter about diet myths and misconceptions, I'd be remiss not to discuss a diet that does work. It's called the Mini-meal Diet, and studies published in the *American Journal of Clinical Nutrition* say it's a smart one.

On this plan you eat mini-meals of 250 to 500 calories per meal. A recent study found that older women (average age 72) who ate these mini-meals burned calories just as fast as younger women (average age 25). When these same older women increased their meals to 1,000 calories, they burned 60 fewer calories than their young counterparts. Over the course of a year, those 60 calories could add up to six pounds and go a long way toward explaining age-related weight gain.

Six Ways to Make Mini-meals Work

1. **Really make these meals mini ones.** Try buying snack-size portions of foods, such as nonfat pudding cups in single-serving sizes, so that you don't overeat. If you buy a family-size box of crackers or shop in the bulk-food aisle, divvy up the large containers into snack-size plastic bags.

2. **Carry your mini-meals with you.** Whole-grain crackers, instant soup cups, low-fat yogurt, baby carrots, and instant oatmeal packets make great at-work mini-meals. Nonperishable items—small boxes of raisins, whole-wheat pretzels, cans of vegetable juice cocktail—can be stashed easily in your briefcase, desk drawer, or car.

3. **Stock your kitchen with items you can quickly turn into mini-meals:** low-fat vanilla yogurt with frozen blueberries, whole-grain cereal with low-fat or soy milk.

4. **If you find that your diet is lacking in certain foods** (dairy foods, fruit, veggies), design your mini-meals to include them.

5. **Make a healthy dessert your family's evening mini-meal.**

6. **Eating out?** Find mini-meals on the menu. If there's an appetizer, there's your mini-meal. If you prefer an entrée, eat only half of it as your mini-meal. Take the rest home for another mini-meal the next day.

A Sample Mini-meal Diet Plan

You can follow a 1,500-calorie diet by eating six 250-calorie mini-meals a day (see a one-day plan below).

7:30 A.M.
1 cup soy protein cereal
1 cup 1% milk
1 cup green tea

9:30 A.M.
1 cup calcium-fortified orange juice
1 slice whole-wheat toast
2 teaspoons whipped reduced-fat butter or low-fat margarine made without trans fats, or 1 teaspoon fruit marmalade

Noon
Veggie burger
Whole-wheat hamburger roll
1 tablespoon mustard
10 sweet red pepper strips
Sliced tomatoes, lettuce

3:30 P.M.
1 cup instant lentil soup

6:30 P.M.
1 cup bulgur
2 cups mixed veggies
2 tablespoons vinaigrette dressing

9 P.M.
1½ ounces reduced-fat cheddar cheese
1 sheet rye crispbread

Sticking with What Works

Mini-meals and diet plans aside, getting and re-maining fit for a lifetime is the best goal of all. Even then it is possible to slip up, but when it happens, you do like Donnie McClurkin advises and get back up. That's what a group of some of the smartest women in the health business did—with a little help from yours truly. As the contributing nutrition editor of *Heart & Soul Magazine*, I counseled the editors during their Get Fit Campaign. Now, you know if anyone knows how to eat to live, it's these women. After all, they're responsible for telling you how to do it each month, right? Well, it didn't work out that way, not at first.

Let me say that the editors of this magazine had the best intentions when they vowed that by hook or crook, they'd lose weight and get fit. Their proclama-tion was admirable. But, sistas, can we talk? I know even health magazine editors occasionally enjoy savor-ing a hunk of chocolate cake or a fried chicken leg, but half of a pizza in one sitting?

When I asked these women to write down every-thing they ate or drank for three days, instead of telling me the truth about what they ate, they recounted how they made "sacrifices" for their families—by taking trips to ice-cream parlors. They told how they crafted complicated schemes to hide giant bags of candy in cellars (and God only knows where else), allegedly to protect their innocent children. They wrote that they just *had* to drink those mega-size orange sodas—you know, to get their vitamin C.

The truth did sneak in here and there. One journal entry simply blared, "I ate all day!" Another: "My hormones are raging, my face is pimple city, and I'm downing a cup of coffee and a doughnut." Another proclaimed angrily, "My mother said the vinegar diet would work; I should trust you over her?"

Truth be told, I knew their pain. Luckily, I knew that as long as the women stayed the course (not the seven courses), they would be okay. And I'm here to say that, by and by, they did.

One finally purged the Pizza Hut phone number from her speed dial. Another boldly kicked her mother out of her house because she was turning her lovely abode into a high-fat snack factory. Still another vowed to give up her favorite hobby: clipping KFC coupons (and not for the coleslaw).

I'm not saying these women didn't get through my tutelage without becoming a bit salty at times. But in the end they were making real commitments—to go meatless once a week, to eat more healthful foods, to drink more water. You see, it turns out the problem wasn't that these good sistas didn't know that eating ribs and chitlins meant there'd be more of them to love. They just love to eat. And that's okay. We're all human, after all. When we fall off the wagon, we get up, dust ourselves off, and keep pressin'.

How We Got Where We Are Today:
The Advice That Backfired

In the 1970s and '80s nutrition experts advised us to cut our consumption of saturated fat and cholesterol to reduce our risk of heart disease. Subsequently, we were subjected to a barrage of nutrition advice designed to help lower the national trend toward obesity and its associated ailments. The message was clear: Fat is bad. We heard this message, and so, too, did the food industry, which began providing a wide array of no-fat, low-fat, reduced-fat, and "lite" products to allow us to eat our cake without eating fat. But if the low-fat message got through, why did it not stem the rising tide of obesity?

With the increasing popularity of diets like the ones I discussed earlier in this chapter, various people have claimed that fat is not the villain. Science writer Gary Taubes wrote an article for *The New York Times Magazine* in 2002 in defense of fat and the Atkins Diet, causing a huge uproar in the nutrition community. It is true that there is conflicting evidence, but I don't agree that the low-fat nutrition messages of the past decades have all been wrong. The facts boil down to this: A group of researchers at Louisiana State University reviewed more than two dozen clinical trials documenting the health benefits of the low-fat diet and found that a 10 percent reduction in dietary fat would net a weight loss of 13 pounds per year. Scores of studies, including the Continuing Survey of Food Intakes by Individuals (CSFII), which examined a random sample of 10,000 American adults, show that people who eat a low-fat diet weigh less than those who eat a high-fat diet. The payoff seemed to be particularly significant for women. The CSFII researchers divided the 10,000 participants into four groups, ranging from those who ate high-carb, low-fat diets to those who ate low-carb, high-fat Atkins-like diets. More than half the women in the low-fat, high-carb diet group had a BMI of less than 25, compared to 45 percent of the women in the Atkins-like group. Generally, males and females in the low-fat, high-carb group consumed an average of 200–300 fewer calories a day than their Atkins cronies.

As we've seen, another group of experts holds that the culprit in your health problems is sugar. The implication is that if we avoid foods with added sugars, we will somehow be able to make a dent in the increasing proportion of obese Americans. But this is not necessarily true, and it's not really the message we want to send.

Seesawing between nutrients as culprits highlights a significant problem with addressing nutritional issues in the United States. Experts oversimplify in order to get their message across. Americans want a magic bullet to good health, and simplifying nutritional issues to bad versus good suggests there is one. But the real message—which is as simple as can be—seems to be getting lost. Eat less, exercise more. That's all there is to it.

Frequently Asked Questions

When it comes to dieting, basically my audience wants to know how to get a great body without doing any work. They want gimmicks and tricks, the kind of thing promised by those dud diets and food fallacies we were talking about earlier, so sometimes I jokingly recommend the "air and water diet"—an absolutely surefire route to weight loss. But seriously, there are no tricks in this business. The only way to lose weight and keep it off is to eat a sensible diet that consists of fewer calories than you burn each day, and to move that body. Fad diets will not get the results you want. So here's more of what people want to know.

Q Dr. Ro: I've been told that I shouldn't eat bananas while trying to lose weight because of their sugar content. Is this true?

A *It is true that bananas, like all carbohydrate foods, do raise blood sugar levels, but they don't force the body to store calories, as you might have been told. Instead, bananas pack a wallop of a nutritional contribution in potassium and magnesium. Both of these minerals are important to muscle contraction, especially important during any workout, because they keep muscles from cramping during your exercise routine. A helpful hint: This sweet fruit makes a good sweetener in cereals and acts as a great substitute for other highly processed sweets, thereby curbing your craving for sweets.*

Q Dr. Ro: As I try to lose weight, I've made changes like eating more vegetables and drinking more water, as you advised, but I have also heard that I shouldn't eat late at night. Is this true?

A *Some research suggests that it's not the time of day we eat that causes us to gain weight, but the amount of food we eat. Other researchers say time of day does matter if you eat high-fat, calorically dense foods, if you are prone to gain weight in your abdominal area (think apple shape), if you are age 40 or over and approaching menopause, and if you are in general prone to overweight—a problem for at least half of all black women. Once you factor in those considerations, eating late may in fact be a factor in weight gain. Here's why: Remember the discussion of pears vs. apples in Secret 2? Well, according to Dr. Pamela Peeke, author of* Fight Fat Over Forty *and an obesity researcher who specializes in stress-hormone-related weight gain, if you consume the bulk of your calories at dinner or in the late evening, the stress hormones that have been building up in your body all during the day are going to create strong cravings for the fats and carbohydrates that fuel the "fight or flight" response, so you'll be likely to eat more. Those same stress hormones, known as cortisols, are also going to stimulate receptors on the fat cells in your abdomen to accept more fat. So if you're eating late, you could be setting yourself up for failure. For this reason, it is probably best to get the bulk of your calories earlier in the day. If you're eating after 6 P.M., Dr. Peeke suggests that you try to limit yourself to vegetables, fruits, and small amounts of lean protein, while avoiding potatoes, pasta, bread, and rice.*

Another reason not to eat too late in the evening is that if you do eat a large quantity of calories within four hours of going to bed, you'll have less of an opportunity to actively burn those calories off than you would in the middle of an active day, so the rate at which they get burned will be much slower. Not to mention the fact that lying down on a full stomach could give you severe indigestion and/or cause a sleepless night.

Q Dr. Ro: What do you think of diet pills and fat burners to lose weight? Do they work?

A *I don't think very much of so-called fat burners at all. Some are more harmful than others. Those with ephedra or ephedrine as the active ingredient have been known to cause heart attack, stroke, seizures, and death; the Food and Drug Administration has restricted fat burners containing ephedra. As for diet pills, sometimes doctors prescribe these for morbidly obese people—those whose weight is 50 to 100 pounds greater than what is considered healthy for them. But even when these are prescribed, a woman should be monitored closely by her physician, and she must learn positive dietary habits that will result in lasting lifestyle changes.*

Secret

Eating Out Will Jam You

If you think you're in a bind at 20 pounds or more over your ideal body weight, and you're eating out three or more times a week, then come talk to me. I know what the problem is. Bottom line, the fast-food joints with their high-fat, supersized meals are going to jam you if you're not careful. So are lots of other restaurants, from the soul food joint on the corner to the most elegant French restaurant with its butter this and cream that—again, if you're not careful. And most of us aren't. Americans, knowing that time is a precious commodity, do everything on the run. We skip breakfast, run errands during lunch hour, and grab something quick before taking our kids to soccer practice at dinnertime. Fast food has replaced baseball as America's national pastime. But all this eating on the go can damage our health.

Our Obsession with Fast Food

Americans shelled out more than $110 billion on burgers, fried chicken, and the like in 2000, up from $6 billion in 1970. And African Americans are no exception; more than 50 percent of us eat out, mostly in the more than 215,000 fast-food restaurants like Burger King, KFC, Taco Bell, and McDonald's. Residents of the United States spend more on fast food each year than they do on movies, books, magazines, newspapers, videos, and compact discs combined. Target Market News, a Chicago-based research company that studies African American consumer trends, found an 18 percent increase between 1998 and 1999 on money spent on fast foods, which tend to be high in fat as well as sodium and sugar, and which constitute most of the food we eat in restaurants. Some of our most popular food buys are hot dogs, white bread, and french fries. Why are African Americans—who earned $500 billion in 2000, enough to make us, collectively, the eleventh richest nation in the world—so enamored with the fast-food lifestyle? The answer is simple and applies to people of all races, ethnicities, and income levels: because fast food is easy. High-fat, high-sugar fast foods are widely available, taste good, and cost less than many healthier foods. Vending machines are ubiquitous. KFC now delivers in some neighborhoods, and most fast-food outlets serve breakfast. Even hospitals—more typically blamed for serving food that is boring and bland, not unhealthy—have gotten into the craze: One study found that a third of the nation's top hospitals now have fast-food franchises in their cafeterias. And most of the fast-food chains do a great job of luring children through their doors with toys, on-site playgrounds and movie tie-ins, spending $3 billion a year on television advertising aimed directly at children. So even adults who might otherwise not be tempted are finding it hard to resist those french fries across the table.

But this obsession with fast and cheap food is one of the culprits in the epidemic of overweight and obesity currently sweeping the country. One supersized fast-food meal can contain a whole day's worth of calories. And even if you choose smaller meals, grabbing a burger and fries or a beef burrito on a daily basis will add the weight quicker than you can say "drive-through." That's what happened to Stacie, a 34-year-old mother and *Heart & Soul* TV viewer who wrote to me after having seen an episode of the show about weight loss strategies. Juggling a husband, a job running a day-care center, two kids, grad school, and all the cooking for a family-owned catering business left little time for preparing healthy meals at home. Six months of nightly fast-food meals and it was Stacie who was supersized, having gained 40 pounds. "I thought I was doing it the right way, ordering the chicken sandwich meal instead of a burger every night," she says now. "But they always asked if I wanted to supersize, and I always said, 'Why not?'" And though she didn't upsize her children's meals, they, too, packed on pounds from their daily fast-food fare; her daughter was wearing a size 10 by the time she was 6 years old, and her son had difficulty fitting into the largest car seat Stacie could find, even though he was only 2.

As Stacie's children show, adults have lots of company in their fast-food dilemma. Many schools have added fast-food outlets to their cafeterias or created fast-food-like items for their cafeteria menus in order to compete with commercial establishments. This craze led former U.S. Surgeon General David Satcher to call for the removal of fast-food items in schools, and there is currently legislation in Congress seeking a ban on junk food in schools.

Check out this table for fat and calorie measurements of some typical fast-food items sold by popular franchises ranging from Arby's to Wendy's. Keep in mind as you read through this list that an average adult's daily calorie intake for weight maintenance is approximately 1,800–2,400 calories, and at the recommended 30 percent of calories from fat, the daily fat allowance for this calorie range is 54 to 72 grams per day.

Table 6-1 Most Popular Fast-Food Meals Calories and Fat Chart

Restaurant / Food	Calories	Fat Grams
Arby's *Regular Roast Beef*	350	16
Blimpie *6-inch Cheese Trio Sub on Wheat*	490	23

Restaurant / Food	Calories	Fat Grams
Boston Market 1/4 White Meat Chicken	140	4
Burger King BK Broiler	317	14
Chick-Fil-A Chicken Sandwich	410	16
Church's Chicken 8-pc. Tender Crunchers	411	15
Dairy Queen Strawberry Blizzard	570	16
Domino's 2 slices Classic Hand-Tossed Cheese Pizza	375	11
Hardee's Hot Dog	450	32
Jack in the Box Sourdough Jack Burger	700	49
KFC 1 drumstick, Original Recipe	140	8
Long John Silver's Regular Battered Fish, 1 pc.	230	13

Restaurant / Food	Calories	Fat Grams
McDonald's		
Big Mac	590	34
Cheeseburger	330	14
Chicken McNuggets 10 pc.	510	33
French fries (large)	540	26
Pizza Hut		
Hand-Tossed Cheese Pizza (1 slice)	240	10
Roy Rogers		
Grilled Chicken Sandwich	340	11
Schlotzsky's		
Deluxe Original Sandwich (small)	693	34
Starbucks		
Blueberry Crumb Cake	800	38
Subway		
6-inch Veggies Delite	230	3
Taco Bell		
1 Soft Taco Supreme, beef	260	14
Wendy's		
8-oz. Chili	200	6
Whataburger		
Double Meat Whataburger	857	48

Upscale Doesn't Mean Healthy

Fast-food joints are not alone in offering high-fat temptations; mid-level restaurants can also be fat traps. Did you visit the salad bar at Ruby Tuesday thinking you were going the healthy route? Well, the spinach, beets, tomatoes, and broccoli are good—but did you add real bacon bits and a lot of shredded cheese? Was the dressing low-fat? How much dressing did you spoon onto your salad? When the waiter brought you another clean plate, did you take your fat-laden salad into a second act? Even when you think you're making healthier choices, the struggle to avoid sugar-laden, high-fat, salty foods can be a dietary nightmare given the amount of food offered at many sit-down restaurants. It seems supersized is not just for fast-food spots anymore. For instance:

❖ The spaghetti and meatball meal at the Olive Garden contains 3 cups of pasta, 7 ounces of meat, and two breadsticks. Between the pasta and the breadsticks (neither of which is made of whole-grain products, by the way), that's 10 of the Food Pyramid's 11 recommended daily grain servings and way more than the 3 to 4 I recommend. Finishing off the 7 ounces of meatballs would completely wipe out your recommended meat servings for the day.

❖ Even if you avoid the burgers and fries at Johnny Rockets, you won't necessarily keep your portion size under control. A tuna salad sandwich contains 4½ ounces of tuna and 3½ ounces of bread. That's two-thirds of your daily protein recommendation and a third of your daily grain portion.

❖ Panda Express's orange-flavored chicken meal includes 8 ounces of chicken and 2 cups of rice. If you're an average-size woman, 9 ounces of protein will satisfy your entire daily protein need. The rice alone accounts for four servings—the number of grains I recommend in my Livin' Healthy Plan for the whole day.

It doesn't get any better at a swanky five-star restaurant, what with cocktails, the bread basket before the meal (usually no whole-grain choices), the main course complete with fat-rich gravies and sauces, and dessert. Did you know that there are steak houses in the Midwest that offer a 48-ounce steak for a meal? That's 3 pounds of meat—enough to feed a family of four all day long!

Test Your Fast-Food Knowledge with the Hidden Fat Traps Quiz

Part of the problem is that we don't know which foods are high in fat. If you really must go the fast-food route, test your fast-food knowledge and learn about the hidden fat traps with the following quiz.

1. Should you pick the Honey Bran Raisin Muffin or the Boston Kreme Donut at Dunkin' Donuts?

*If you chose the muffin, which certainly **sounds** healthier, you're wrong: It's loaded with 490 calories and 14 grams of fat, while the Boston Kreme Donut has 240* calories and 9 grams of fat. Better still—order a whole-grain bagel (a small one has 350 calories, 4.5 fat grams), eat only half of it, and save the other half for the next day.

2. Are the Chicken McNuggets or the hamburger the better choice at McDonald's?

At 280 calories and with 10 grams of fat, the small plain hamburger wins hands down, compared to the high-fat 10 piece McNuggets, which weighs in at 510 calories and 33 grams of fat. If you like chicken and happen to be dining under the golden arches, I suggest opting for the Grilled Chicken Caesar Salad, which is a pretty smart choice at a mere 210 calories and 7 grams of fat. Top it with the 30-calorie, fat-free Herb Vinaigrette, and you'll be in McHeaven.

3. Got a hankerin' for pizza? Which is the best choice at Pizza Hut, the Pepperoni Hand Tossed or the Veggie Lover's Stuffed Crust Pizza?

Surprise—the Pepperoni Hand Tossed (280 calories, 18 grams of fat per slice) is actually better than the Veggie Lover's Stuffed Crust Pizza (340 calories, 14 grams of fat per slice). Sure, the veggies are good, but they're sitting atop a mountain of cheese. Best of all is the Veggie Lover's Hand Tossed Pizza (220 calories, 8 grams of fat per slice).

4. When you stop for breakfast at McDonald's, should you have the bacon, egg, and cheese biscuit or the Egg McMuffin?

Go for the McMuffin. It contains 300 calories and 12 grams of fat. The bacon, egg, and cheese biscuit, on the *other hand, is loaded with 480 calories and 31 grams of fat.*

5. Which should you opt for, the BK Fish Filet Sandwich or the Whopper hamburger at Burger King?

You probably think fish is the way to go for a healthy fast-food meal. Think again. Burger King's Whopper Jr. comes in at 397 calories and 22 grams of fat. The BK Fish Filet Sandwich contains 446 calories and 22 grams of fat.

6. Got a craving for chicken? How about the chicken pot pie at Kentucky Fried?

There are healthy choices at KFC, but the chunky chicken pot pie (770 calories, 40 grams of fat) is not among them—it's loaded with cream sauce and fat. Also avoid the Triple Crunch Sandwich (540 calories and 26 grams of fat), which is fried. Your best choice is the Tender Roast Chicken Sandwich—only 260 calories and 5 grams of fat if you get it without sauce.

7. If you've really got a jones for something sweet, is there anything in the fast-food lane that isn't loaded with fat?

Choose a Mrs. Fields apple bran muffin. It's pretty hefty in the calorie count at 340, but it contains only 2.5 grams of fat. And high calorie count and all, it's head and shoulders above the sticky bun (880 calories, 34 grams of fat).

8. Beans are lighter than beef, right?

Not exactly. Taco Bell's beef soft taco has 210 calories and 10 grams of fat. The bean burrito has 370 calories and 10 grams of fat.

Other Hidden Highs

Even when we try to avoid the fast-food craze by preparing quick frozen meals at home, we can still run into problems. Believe me, I know it's tempting: Frozen entrées are a quick and easy answer to "What's for dinner?" and there are no pots and pans to clean up after the meal is complete. Pop your meal in the microwave (roughly 8 in 10 homes now own one) and you're eating. But many if not most frozen meals have one drawback: high salt levels.

Just because the label says low fat doesn't mean a food is low in sodium. Keep these numbers in mind when choosing: Food is considered low in sodium if it has 140 milligrams or less of sodium per serving. In general you should try not to have more than 2,400 milligrams of sodium each day, which doesn't sound too hard. But in fact it's easier said than done, because although you might not be shaking salt anymore, what you may not know is that most of the sodium in our diets doesn't come from the salt shaker; nearly 75 percent of our sodium comes in the form of processed foods. Even foods that you don't think of as salty, such as instant pudding, contain sodium, usually about 500 milligrams per serving. And most frozen foods—even the healthy versions—have a high sodium content. Entrée-only frozen meals, which come with no added veggies or side dishes, are especially guilty of this. Also note that frozen breakfast entrées tend to be very salty.

Take a look at the sodium content of some popular choices.

Table 6-2 High-Sodium Frozen Meals

Brand / Entrée	Sodium (milligrams)
Armour Classics Light *Chicken à la King*	630
Budget Gourmet Light *Glazed Turkey*	760
Dining Light *Fettuccini with Broccoli*	1,020
Healthy Choice *Shrimp Creole*	560
Lean Cuisine *Filet of Fish Divan*	750
Le Menu *Chicken Kiev*	780
Stouffer's *Pasta Primavera*	580
Tyson *Peking Chicken*	860
Weight Watchers *Chicken Divan Baked Potato*	730

To limit your sodium intake, keep the following in mind:

❖ Limit your use of salty condiments (olives, pickles, soy sauce, steak sauce).
❖ Use herbs and spices instead of salt when you cook. Good ones to try include cumin, dill, fresh garlic or garlic powder, lemon, mustard, and onion.
❖ Substitute plain or oven-roasted meats for cured or smoked meats.
❖ Check your food labels for sodium content.

Best Fast-Food Bets

Does all this bad fast-food news mean you have to cross Taco Bell and KFC off your list altogether? No. Some fast-food places have started catering to their customers' needs with healthier menu items. Subway has seven 6-inch sub sandwiches that come in at less than 325 calories (remember the Jared commercials?). And all of them have 6 grams of fat or less. Wendy's new Garden Sensations salad line has a Mandarin Chicken Salad with 150 calories and only 1.5 grams of fat. Taco Bell switched from lard to corn oil, and most other fast-food chains have also made the switch to 100 percent vegetable shortening. You can also build a healthier fast-food restaurant meal by keeping these tips in mind:

❖ Go for salads. Just refrain from piling on the high-fat, high-sodium salad companions such as eggs, bacon bits, cheese, and mounds of fat-laden dressing.

❖ Stick to charbroiled and roasted sandwiches.

❖ Choose diet sodas or tea instead of regular sodas.

❖ Try frozen yogurt desserts instead of ice cream.

❖ Avoid deep-dish pan pizzas, and choose plain thin-crust or veggie pizzas instead. Ask for more vegetables and half the cheese when you place your order.

❖ Use fruit marmalade or jam on your bread instead of margarine or butter.

Beware of Healthy-Sounding Foods

Don't let the name of an entrée fool you into thinking you're making a healthy choice. Just because it's chicken, fish, or vegetables doesn't mean it's healthy. Make a point of knowing how a food is prepared—whether it's fried (unhealthy) or broiled (more likely to be healthy), for example—and what's on top of it. Taco Bell's Taco Salad has a whopping 790 calories, while McDonald's Chef Salad (with Thousand Island Dressing) has 620 calories. A Burger King Chicken Whopper has 590 calories, and Wendy's chicken club sandwich has 470 calories. The Baked Alaskan Salmon Platter at Long John Silver's has 690 calories.

Staying the Course

Healthy eating out doesn't mean you can't have any of your favorite foods. You just have to know how to choose healthy versions of those foods.

Breakfast

Off the chain (smart choices): pancakes (hold the butter), fresh fruit, cereal, whole-wheat toast, vegetable juice, fruit juice

Slow your roll (go easy choices): bacon, hash browns, sausage, omelets, breakfast sandwiches

Appetizer

Off the chain (smart choices): steamed veggies, dinner salads, seafood cocktails, steamed seafood

Slow your roll (go easy choices): fried veggies or cheese, potato skins, tortilla chips

Bread

Off the chain (smart choices): whole-grain breads, flat breads

Slow your roll (go easy choices): biscuits, croissants, muffins

Salad

Off the chain (smart choices): lemon wedges,
gourmet vinegar, reduced-calorie or fat-free
dressings

Slow your roll (go easy choices): avocado, bacon
bits, cheese, olives, regular dressings

Entrée

Off the chain (smart choices): any tofu, textured
vegetable protein, fish, turkey, chicken, small
portion of lean beef, or veal that is steamed,
grilled, baked, or broiled, topped with veggies
when and where possible; beans prepared
without cheese or cream sauces

Slow your roll (go easy choices): potpies, quiches,
cheese-based items, fried foods, large portions

Beverage

Off the chain (smart choices): water, fruit juice
spritzer (a splash of fruit juice in a glass of
seltzer or club soda), nonfat or low-fat milk,
juice, tea

Slow your roll (go easy choices): sodas, milk
shakes (although McDonald's milk shakes are
low in fat, with less than 2 grams of fat per
shake)

Special beverage note #1: Think of water as the
liquid of your life. It's calorie-free and makes
you less likely to overeat. That's why sipping

water before, during, and after meals is a good addition to the successful dieter's bag of tricks. It fills the belly faster and kills hunger pangs. Two glasses of water after a meal help wash away excess sodium, especially if you've dipped into a fast-food joint. And there's an added benefit: Not only does drinking water bathe cells and lubricate your skin, but you'll also be happy to know that it speeds up your metabolism. You'll know you're drinking enough water if your urine is clear and colorless all day.

Special beverage note #2: Tea, by all accounts, is really good for you. A recent study found that a serving of black tea had more antioxidants—crucial to your body's defense against heart disease and cancer—than a serving of broccoli or carrots.

Dessert

Off the chain (smart choices): angel food cake, fresh berries, ices, nonfat frozen yogurt, sorbet

Slow your roll (go easy choices): cake, cookies, ice cream, doughnuts, pie

All-You-Can-Eat Buffets

Off the chain (smart choices): raw fruits and veggies, small plates, tiny portions

Slow your roll (go easy choices): casseroles,

multiple trips to the buffet table, industrial-size portions

Eating When It's a Family Affair

The Sunday dinners you have with your family may remind you of the ones you saw in the movie *Soul Food*. Wherever your family gatherings take place, you may find that you're not getting the support you need for your new health style from family members. So to keep to your plan, bring along a dish that you've prepared using ingredients that you have modified for healthy eating. It might be a sweet potato casserole, but your sweet potatoes will be light on the fat and sugar, and if you do it right, they'll ask *you* for the recipe. (If you don't have any ideas of your own, check out my recipe for sweet potatoes with apples and raisins in Secret 10.) Without being preachy, use the opportunity to enlighten family members about small lifestyle changes, and encourage them to join you in the fight for better health. Explain that as a family, it's a good thing for the whole clan. When your idea catches on, try family cook-offs, pitting the elders against the upstarts to show off their stuff in the kitchen—this time in a healthier fashion.

Eating at the Office

First things first: Don't skip meals. Start your day with a good breakfast at home, and don't skimp on lunch because you're too busy to eat. Next, step away from the vending machines. They won't give you balanced nutrition, and they almost always offer choices that are less than healthful. In fact, it is usually easier on the pocketbook and easier on your calorie and fat budget to take control by bringing your own lunch. Fill your lunch bag with a nutritious survival kit, much like you would if you were taking a trip on a plane. That means packing fresh veggies and fruit and, if you have them, some leftovers from last night's dinner. A quick and easy way to assemble a meal from leftovers is to start with a small portion of meat, say from a roasted chicken left over from Sunday's dinner. That chicken can be made into sandwiches using whole-wheat bread topped with a few sprouts, lettuce leaves, and cucumber slices. Add a small portion of baby carrots, an apple, and a bottle of water, and that, my sista, is lunch. Another portion of that leftover chicken can be topped with fat-free salsa (think disease-fighting lycopene) and served with a salad, and again you've got lunch. The rest of the chicken you can toss with a tarragon-mustard dressing made with non-fat yogurt as the basis for a healthful chicken salad to which your choice of extras can be added—tomatoes, diced cucumbers, maybe even a few walnuts. Serve over fresh watercress or endive and you have yet another delicious lunch.

The trick is to keep foods on hand that you can assemble a meal from, even if you don't consider yourself a cook. If properly planned, packing your own lunch takes little time, makes for convenient eating, and helps you to control the nutritional value of your food choices. Other lunchable choices are healthful frozen meals if your office has a microwave (stick

to those with 9 grams of fat or less per serving), soy
shakes, or drained vacuum-packed tuna with a sliced
tomato and whole-wheat crackers.

Eating Around the World

Ordering ethnic food requires that you pay a little
more attention to what's in the food and how it's
cooked. This may mean you have to ask the waiter or
the chef how your meal is prepared.

Soul Food

Most African Americans know exactly where to
find the best soul food restaurant in town; in D.C.,
where I live, it's the Florida Avenue Grill. But when
you eat there, avoid the smothered chicken, chicken-
fried steak, macaroni and cheese, and mashed potatoes
with gravy. Instead, opt for string beans, collards, and
corn bread (without butter). And remember: Don't be
afraid to ask how the food is prepared. Since any soul
food restaurant will typically prepare foods the traditional way, it is very difficult to control anything but
portions. So if you've just got to have one of the high-
calorie entrées, eat half a portion.

Caribbean

To go healthy in a Caribbean restaurant, choose the
jerk chicken, vegetable patties, grilled snapper, pepper-
pot, roti, conch, and other salads. Curried shrimp is
also a good bet, but always ask if they've prepared it
(or any of your favorites) using coconut milk, palm oil,
or palm kernel oil, all of which you want to avoid. You

can often get steamed fish dishes in Caribbean restaurants, so look the menu over carefully before making your selections.

African

I said it before, and I'll say it again here: Made with plenty of fresh veggies, African food can be healthy if it's prepared properly. Your best bets at that new African restaurant downtown are couscous, leafy green vegetables, grilled fish, boiled plantain, and poulet yassa (chicken marinated in an onion-lemon-mustard mix). Note: Many African dishes use peanut oil, which is on a par with olive oil on a health scale, but should be avoided by people with peanut allergies because it can cause very serious reactions. Also avoid palm oil and palm kernel oil, both of which are saturated fats and raise cholesterol levels.

Mexican

Before you begin the meal, hold the chips (a basket is worth 645 calories and 34 grams of fat). Soft corn tortillas, salsas or picante sauces, rice and black beans (prepared without lard or fat), and spicy or grilled chicken dishes make good choices. Hold the cheese, sour cream, refried beans, chimichangas, chiles rellenos, and—although it counts as a smart choice for a monounsaturated fat—go easy on the guacamole. The sour cream and guacamole alone can rack up an extra 24 grams of fat. Grilled chicken fajitas are good bets for nutrition and flavor. Try anything in the veracruz style, which in Mexican cuisine means a sauce made with tomatoes, onions, and chiles.

Chinese

There's a Chinese food restaurant on nearly every corner in our neighborhoods. But contrary to popular opinion in the black community, Chinese isn't synonymous with healthy and low-fat. The healthiest items on the menu include hot and sour soup (often made with tofu), spicy green beans, moo shu shrimp, vegetable lo mein, shrimp with broccoli, and yu hsiang eggplant. Other good bets are Szechwan shrimp, steamed chicken, even duck with hoisin sauce. Choose dishes that have been made without MSG (monosodium glutamate), a very high-sodium flavor enhancer. Ask the waiter or chef to make recommendations of menu items that are steamed, poached, roasted, or barbecued. Avoid stir-fried, deep-fried, or "crispy" entrées, because most are made with as much fat as found in 16 strips of bacon (that's 56 grams, or 4 tablespoons of oil). And always opt for steamed rice rather than fried rice. For dessert, stick with the fortune cookie and have the orange wedges or pineapple pieces, typically offered free of charge to patrons at the end of the meal. The fruit is a fat-free choice, with only about 25 calories.

Italian

If it hasn't been Americanized, this can be very healthy eating. In fact, that's what the Mediterranean diet is all about—health! Grilled vegetables and green salads are good choices. For meats or protein, choose veal, chicken, fish prepared with garlic and olive oil, minestrone, or white beans (sometimes called cannelini beans). Think RED (as in tomato) when it comes to sauce. Whole-grain couscous and polenta make low-fat, high-fiber side dishes. Choose sun-dried or crushed tomato dishes, and meat or fish that is grilled, lightly sautéed, or prepared with lemon—"piccata." But piccata may include lots of butter or olive oil, so ask before ordering. Ordering half portions of pasta and entrées is very easy to do at many Italian restaurants, and other restaurants will sometimes accommodate this request as well. But avoid eggplant parmigiana, fettuccini alfredo, lasagna, garlic bread, and other dishes heavy on cream, eggs, butter, or cheese. In general you should go easy on the cheese. You can eat 1 cup of pasta and ½ cup of marinara sauce with 1 tablespoon of cheese on top and it'll cost you no more than 300 calories and 6 grams of fat.

In *all* restaurants of *any* ethnicity you should ask your waiter how the food is prepared before you order. Many restaurants will adapt dishes to your preference—by serving sauce on the side, for example, or sautéing your food choice with less butter or oil.

Tips to Get You Through the Eating-Out Maze

Many people get discouraged by the challenge of restaurant eating when they are trying to improve their diets, but there are ways to eat out and do so in a healthful manner. Try these tips:

❖ Select foods that are steamed, broiled, grilled, roasted, or baked instead of fried or sautéed.
❖ Don't go to dinner on an empty stomach. It

might seem like common sense, but it bears saying: If you're starving, you're more likely to pile your plate high.

❖ Share an entrée with someone else.

❖ Try an appetizer as an entrée.

❖ Order à la carte, because that way you'll be getting only the foods you really want, instead of a whole plateful of foods that you may end up eating just because they're there in front of you.

❖ Ask for a take-away (doggy) bag *before* you eat, and request that part of the meal be put away immediately, to take home for later. That way you won't have to exercise any willpower in order to be sure that you eat only a half portion.

❖ Eat slowly. It takes roughly 20 minutes for your brain to get the message that you're full. Relax, enjoy the company of your guests, and concentrate more on the fellowship and social aspects of the meal.

❖ Stop eating the minute you feel full. You should be satisfied, not stuffed.

❖ Ask for your salad dressing on the side. Salads such as Caesar salad, which come with dressings already added, are not the best choice.

❖ Limit your alcohol intake. It may seem like a small drink, but a 4½-ounce piña colada contains 262 calories; a 2½-ounce martini has 156 calories.

❖ Stay away from mayonnaise and sauces. Ask for mustard, relish, or cranberry sauce, or simply more lettuce, sprouts, or tomatoes instead. If the dish comes with a sauce, ask for it to be served on the side, then use a small amount of the sauce for "taste" rather than having excess amounts of fat. Red sauces, such as tomato sauce and salsa, are usually lower in fat than oily or creamy sauces.

❖ Avoid cheese. Although rich in calcium, cheese is chock-full of cholesterol and saturated fat. Few restaurants prepare food using low-fat cheeses.

❖ Eat whole-wheat dinner rolls without the butter. It is likely that the rest of the meal will have some fat already added, so you don't need the butter. If a mixture of oil and balsamic vinegar is provided as a dip for bread, ask for straight balsamic vinegar.

❖ A salad or vegetable plate is a better appetizer than soup or other mixed dish, where it's difficult to determine the fat content of the item.

❖ Avoid buffets, all-you-can-eat menus, or smorgasbords; the temptation to eat all you can or to try some of each item can overwhelm your efforts to make good choices.

❖ If you order pasta, avoid filled or stuffed pastas such as ravioli, tortellini, or wontons.

❖ A baked potato or plain rice is lower in fat than fried or mashed potatoes or rice pilaf.

❖ Go small. A regular-size burger or roast beef sandwich provides two servings of grains and

3 ounces of protein, just the right amount for a meal.

✤ Roast beef and turkey are better choices than burgers.

✤ Choose low-fat desserts—sorbet, fruit cup, frozen yogurt, or gelatin. If you simply must have the traditional high-fat dessert such as the huge double-chocolate brownie topped with a scoop of vanilla bean ice cream, split it with a companion.

✤ Choose one "splurge" food per meal, then finish off your meal with a healthful favorite. That's called balance!

On the Road (or in the Skies) Again

As many of you will remember, back in the day, we used to take along little brown bags full of food any time we made a road trip. Those sacks were filled with souse (hog's head cheese), potted meat, and greasy fried chicken. You can probably still picture (and smell) those brown, grease-spotted sacks that went with you to Big Mama's house down South. We ate this way on the road because racism was so pervasive then that it prevented black folks from stopping at roadside diners for a bite to eat. Even though those days are gone now and there's been a huge prolifera- tion of fast-food restaurants, small diners, and casual eateries lining the highways and welcoming all, we still carry that portable greasy-spoon meal—mainly out of habit. I have to admit that eating healthy on the road is a challenge. But if you'll follow my suggestions above for making good choices in fast food and other restaurants, you should be able to eat sensibly as well as inexpensively.

Planes: The Waiting Game

Most airports haven't provided food services that cater to healthful eating habits. If your flight is delayed or canceled and you want to eat a meal, often the only thing available is fast food. On a recent layover in Chicago, I waited just outside my designated gate for nearly two hours. Due to increased security measures, passengers headed to Washington, D.C., weren't allowed to sit in the gate area until just prior to boarding the flight. Once through security, the only food options near the gate area were foot-long hot dogs, a deep-dish pizzeria, a bar, McDonald's, Mrs. Fields Cookies, and a candy stand. Fortunately, I had a couple of boxes of raisins and an apple stashed in my purse. Not so for the other passengers; McDonald's did a brisk business that day.

Don't get caught in this trap if you get stuck in an airport. Eating out of boredom, sipping cocktails at the bar, and sampling the candy will certainly crash-land your diet.

Even with these seemingly impossible choices, there are options. Most of the nation's largest and busiest airports offer fresh fruit and fruit juices, salads, pretzels, and low-fat or nonfat yogurt. Even in fast-food restaurants, you don't necessarily have to be held hostage. Take a walk first to explore your options. The walk will do your body good, and it'll give you time to make an

Holiday Noshing

The holidays are here, and you know how black folks like to celebrate! The good news: All those parties and open houses can make meal planning unnecessary during this time of year. The bad news: You're only a few meatballs, cheese platters, chips, and rolls away from blowing your healthy meal plan. Here's a tip to keep in mind: Single-ingredient items—shrimp, skewered chicken breasts, raw vegetables—are less likely to harbor hidden calories than meatballs or spinach-cheese puffs.

Recent reports have found that we don't gain as much during the holiday season as previously thought, putting on only about a pound instead of five pounds. But that same research found that once we add that pound, we're more likely to keep it on. Even assuming that's the only weight we gain each year, that's an extra 10 pounds each decade!

That last cookie on the plate may be calling your name like the Sirens of Greek mythology, but you can avoid it. Here are a few tips:

❖ Just as you shouldn't go to a restaurant or the grocery store while you're starving, you shouldn't attend a holiday party on an empty stomach, either. Eat something light before you go.

❖ Wear something snug to your holiday party as a reminder not to overindulge.

continued

- ❖ Don't stand next to the food table.
- ❖ Increase your activity level during the holidays. If you get into the habit of taking a brisk walk every day in December, the healthy habit may carry over into the new year.
- ❖ Dip with vegetables, not chips.

informed decision. This will also prevent the temptation to grab something, anything, just because it's available.

Better yet, plan ahead. Pack survival snacks: dried and fresh fruits, nuts, protein bars, whole-grain crackers, single-serving boxes of whole-grain cereal, soy nuts, ostrich sticks (which resemble Slim Jim beef sticks), and dried and fresh vegetables.

To really maximize the health benefits you get from making wise food choices, keep yourself in motion by skipping the people mover. You'll burn calories by walking whenever and wherever possible. Given the distances that have to be traveled as you make your way through the terminals of a typical big-city airport, you could easily get a day's worth of walking in if you decided to avoid the easy way.

Best Bets in the Air

Many airlines have specialty meals—religious, diabetic, low-sodium, vegetarian. You just have to remember to preorder them. Most airlines require between 6 and 24 hours' notice. Otherwise you'll get stuck eating those regular in-flight meals, which can easily run you 600 calories (a Sky Chefs roasted chicken meal, which has roasted chicken, rice pilaf, green beans, green salad with vinegar and oil dressing, 2 slices whole-wheat bread, 1 pat margarine, and shortbread cookies, contains 738 calories and 34 grams of fat). The small snack packs aren't much better; a bag of peanuts is roughly 166 calories, and salty, to boot!

If you aren't able to order a specialty meal, there are things you can do to lessen the hit on your diet. Use only half the packet of salad dressing, omit the margarine, and don't eat the cookies. You'll save 155 calories. If you're flying during a breakfast meal, pass on the hot meal and opt for cold cereal, which usually comes with fresh fruit and low-fat or nonfat milk. Drink water instead of soda or alcoholic beverages, and not just because of the calories. The low humidity and recirculating air in the pressurized cabin make air travel a dehydrating experience, so it's best to go easy on alcohol as well as caffeine, since both further dehydrate you.

Trains: Best Bets in the Station

Train stations, like airports, tend to be crowded with fast-food places and snack carts. But like airports, they also usually have some fresh fruit, yogurt, salads, maybe even air-popped popcorn for sale.

Best Bets on the Tracks

The café car is open for business—and full of fat-laden foods such as hot dogs, sodas, chips, and cookies. If you have to eat there, choose deli-style sandwiches and small salads. Always ask for more vegetables to be added, such as lettuce, tomato, onions, bell peppers, carrots, and sprouts. Get your condiments on the side. But my favorite option is always to bring your own healthful snacks.

Frequently Asked Questions

Q Dr. Ro: I'm a 20-year-old college student with few options for food, and there's no fresh fruit in the café. Help!

A *College life can be a blast, yet you have challenges that many of us do not. For one, funds are usually limited, and often the food available to you in the dorm or on campus is, too. So what do you do? You stop by the nearest fast-food joint to grab something, anything, and since you want to make your buck go as far as it can, and because you're not sure when you'll eat again, you go the supersize route. Right? Well, listen up. Supersizing your way through school will do more than fill and swell your belly; it'll help you dig yourself an early grave through a tunnel of obesity and overweight. Larger portions of high-fat, high-sodium food, on top of the sedentary lifestyle of our computer-hugging, book-reading, and paper-writing students, explains why so many of you are overweight and even obese. But you're looking for a solution, so I won't beat you over the head with what you probably already know. Here are a few helpful hints to get you through the college years with fewer inches around your waist.*

First, stock your cabinets with healthy foods you can eat on the run, on the way to class, in student meetings, or at Greek functions. Whatever your daily routine, these are must-haves to keep with you or in your room or apartment. Vacuum-packed tuna in a foil package travels easily. It's a good low-fat protein source and can be eaten plain or mixed with packets of reduced-fat mayo or mustard, which is naturally fat-free. An even easier alternative is the lunch-on-the-run canned tuna meal that comes complete with whole-wheat crackers, reduced-fat mayo, and a packet of relish. Other handy must-haves are soy-based crunchy cereal (I like Kashi Go Lean Crunch); Kellogg's Smart Start; fresh vegetables (carrots, tomatoes, celery, broccoli, bell peppers, and romaine lettuce, for easy salads or just to munch on); marinated, grilled, or roasted veggies (available at most grocery deli counters); and fresh apples, pears, oranges, peaches, plums, or grapefruit. There's also dried fruit like cranberries, cran-raisins, apricots, and peaches, although they contain more sugar than their fresh counterparts. A lot of common grocery stores now carry dried veggies to snack on (they're great in place of chips and cheese curls). For protein, peanut butter is good to keep on hand; spread it thinly—because of its high fat content—on cucumber slices and fresh fruit or make sandwiches with it. Though slightly lower in protein than peanut butter, hummus, a Mediterranean spread made of chickpeas, is a good choice, too. Spread it on crackers or fresh veggies for an extra nutritional punch. Also try soy nuts; they're high in protein and crunchy, like your favorite salty snack, only healthier.

Most of you have refrigerators in your rooms, so keep skim or low-fat milk on hand to have with cereal in the morning or afternoon. One deli-counter rotisserie chicken *can get you through almost an entire week. Make sandwiches with part of it; add 2 ounces of chopped chicken to a serving of Oodles of Noodles, top it off with a little diced celery, spring onion, and carrot, skip the seasoning packet, add a splash of low-fat soy sauce or a tablespoon of hoisin sauce, and you've got a gourmet meal. If you're in the mood for a salad, add a 2-ounce serving of chicken to a heaping bowl of salad greens, toss with a couple of tablespoons of fat-free Caesar salad dressing, and you've made yourself a chicken Caesar salad. And you thought you couldn't cook.*

Contents of an On-Campus Survival Kit for the Kitchen:

- ✔ Fresh fruit
- ✔ Fresh vegetables
- ✔ Roasted deli chicken
- ✔ Chinese noodles
- ✔ Kashi Go Lean Crunch cereal or Kellogg's Smart Start
- ✔ Dried soy nuts
- ✔ Reduced-fat or skim milk
- ✔ Fruit juice
- ✔ Canned fruit
- ✔ Dried fruit
- ✔ Vacuum-packed or canned tuna
- ✔ Reduced-fat mayo or mustard
- ✔ Reduced-sodium soy sauce
- ✔ Hoisin sauce
- ✔ Peanut butter
- ✔ Whole-wheat crackers

Q Dr. Ro: There is always food in my office. If it isn't someone's birthday or retirement party, we're toasting a new baby or an engagement. I know most of the food at these gatherings isn't healthy, but I can't always refuse to eat. What should I do?

A *Set a good example by bringing something healthy—a fresh fruit or vegetable platter— to the office potluck. Take only small portions of foods brought by your co-workers. Throw away your plate once you have finished the first helping in order to resist the temptation of seconds or (yikes!) thirds.*

Secret 7

Heart Disease Begins at Six

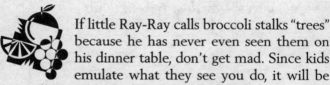 If little Ray-Ray calls broccoli stalks "trees" because he has never even seen them on his dinner table, don't get mad. Since kids emulate what they see you do, it will be virtually impossible to get your brood to eat their vegetables if you never eat any yourself. The fact is, while two-thirds of American adults are overweight, and over half of African American women are, too, our children are not far behind. Childhood obesity has doubled in the last 20 years, with one in four, or a quarter, of American children considered obese. As with almost every epidemic and disease, the numbers are worse for black youth: Nearly 22 percent of African American children are obese.

Not only are more children overweight, but those who are weigh in at 20 to 30 percent heavier than their overweight cousins from 10 years ago. These disturbing trends are reflected in a national survey that followed 8,270 U.S. children between the ages of 4 and 12 from

1986 to 1998. At the beginning of the study about 20 percent of black and white children alike had BMIs greater than what had been the 85th percentile for children in their age and gender group in the 1960s—which is the cutoff now used to identify children who are overweight or at risk of being overweight. But by the end of the study, the percentage of black children with BMIs at or above the 85th percentile had increased to 38 percent, while the percentage of white children at that level or higher had increased only to 26 percent. The fact that the number of children who are overweight or at risk of being overweight keeps increasing, especially among African Americans (and also Hispanics), is very alarming. According to government estimates, some 6 million children are fat enough that their health is at stake; another 5 million are waiting to slide down the slippery slope. That's one child in three who is either overweight or in danger of becoming so.

This is ridiculous! Endangering our own adult lives is bad enough. To carry the obesity epidemic over into the next generation is tragic, and since it is clearly a preventable problem, we must commit ourselves to ending it.

The explosion in the numbers of overweight and obese children can at least in part be attributed to the fact that we have replaced home cooking with fast food in our hustle-and-bustle society. The startling revelation that kids spend on average 24 to 40 hours a week in front of a television set, depending on their age group, surely accounts for much of the rest of this epidemic, since time spent in front of a TV is time not spent running, jumping rope, or throwing balls on the basketball court. Recent research found that children from low-income families with a television in the bedroom watch five more hours of TV each week than their peers without a television in the bedroom. These same kids, says the study, are 40 percent more likely than their peers to be overweight. Another study found that the rate of obesity increases 2 percent for each hour of TV a child watches each day.

But the problem doesn't stop at a particular income level. If they are kids from middle- or upper-class families with resources, they are likely to spend an inordinate amount of time in front of a computer screen or playing video games. Since physical education has been whittled down to little or nothing in many public schools and there has been a sharp decline in youth sports participation, our kids are essentially out of luck when it comes to having either the opportunity for physical exercise or any kind of school or community encouragement for planned sports activities. In fact, fewer than half of U.S. schoolchildren participate in daily physical education. All this is happening at the same time as fast-food and soda consumption within school walls is increasing. Though some school districts have decided to ban the sale of soft drinks on school campuses, far too few schools have established such a sensible policy. So it's really up to us to get our kids moving and to see to it that their meals are nutritionally sound.

BMI Charts for Kids

Until recently, childhood obesity was rare and physicians and other experts really didn't track it. Determining BMIs, the height-to-weight ratio used to assess adult weight that we discussed in detail in Secret 2, was deemed unnecessary, silly even, for children, whose bodies are still growing. And if BMIs were calculated, the criteria for overweight were the same for children as for adults. Now that mind-set has changed. The Centers for Disease Control recently published new charts that create a different way of using BMIs to assess children, which includes everyone between ages 2 and 20. Unlike the adult charts, which classify all people of both sexes and all ages as overweight if they have a BMI over 25 or obese if their BMI is over 30, the childhood charts that define overweight and obesity take both age and gender into account. And in order to allow for "baby fat" and for the normal weight gain that precedes a child's growth spurts, the new charts use a very broad definition of what amounts to a healthy weight for children. For example, to be considered at risk of becoming too heavy (having a BMI over what had been the 85th percentile for girls her age in the 1960s), a 17-year-old girl standing 5 feet 4 inches would have to weigh 145 pounds or more. Only after hitting 170 pounds (the weight cutoff for the 95th percentile) would she be classified as actually overweight. But at that weight, she is considered likely to remain overweight as an adult and be at risk of cardiovascular disease. More and more pediatricians are now using the BMI charts that were created by the CDC, so if you're concerned about whether your child is overweight, ask.

Early Death Warrants

Know this: Fat kids will more than likely become fat adults. Studies show that 70 to 80 percent of kids who are overweight at age 10 to 13 will be overweight or obese as adults. Children who are obese at age 6 have a 50 percent chance of being obese adults. The reason for this is probably the same reason that overweight or obese adults tend to stay that way. It's very hard to change habits and lose weight. And for the record, obesity breeds disease, even in children. Researchers who looked at 6- and 7-year-old cadavers were able to see that fatty streaks had already begun to form in their tiny arteries, and other researchers have found signs of hardening of the arteries, or atherosclerosis, in children as young as 3. Overweight children tend to have readings in the highest levels of the normal ranges for their blood sugar, blood pressure, and blood fats. All this evidence suggests that heart disease and some of its risk factors, like high blood pressure, get their start long before adulthood.

One of the primary causes of the risk factors for heart and circulatory diseases as well as diabetes is a poor diet. A diet that is high in sugar, sodium, and fat and low in fiber—in other words, a typical fast-food diet—offers little nutritional benefit and can do a lot of damage to your child's health. There's nothing theoretical about these dangers. Nutritionists and physicians have reported that their youthful patients are being diagnosed in alarming numbers with high cholesterol; high blood pressure (obese children are more than twice as likely to develop hypertension); fatty liver, a precursor to cirrhosis; obstructive sleep apnea, a condition in which excess flesh around the throat blocks the airway, causing loud snoring and a chronic lack of oxygen that can damage the heart and lungs; type II diabetes (one in four overweight children shows signs of the disease); and a myriad of other diseases, including some cancers, that used to be associated only with adults. As recently as 1990, less than 4 percent of children with diabetes had type II. Now the American Diabetes Association reports that as many as 45 percent of newly diagnosed cases of diabetes in children are type II. That is a truly shocking increase, especially when you consider that it is largely preventable.

There's also some alarming evidence from a recent Yale University study that tested kids for evidence of impaired glucose tolerance, one of the precursors of type II diabetes. (Impaired glucose tolerance means that the body is not able to process food properly and the sugar levels in the blood rise higher than normal after eating, but not high enough to constitute a diagnosis of diabetes.) Of kids age 4 to 10 in the study, 25 percent had impaired glucose tolerance, indicating that this startling epidemic of cases of type II diabetes in children could grow even more widespread. The study also found that 4 percent of the obese adolescents already had type II diabetes, of which neither they nor their parents were aware. Since many children are not routinely tested for diabetes, pediatricians worry that as alarming as the statistics regarding type II diabetes are, in reality they are probably even worse than we know.

The physical implications of being overweight and obese are bad enough for your kids, but what about the emotional toll? Children can be brutally honest and often far more critical than adults. They can hurt the very fragile feelings of your precious one by name-calling, teasing, and harmful chatter. Of course, the primary concern here should be your child's health, but consider that her health extends beyond her vital organs to her very self-image and feelings of self-worth. Moreover, if there are bullies in the school-yard—and there usually are—feelings may not be the only things that get hurt, even in the short term.

Nicole's Story: ✦ I met Michelle after she heard me give a speech during my Tampax Total You Tour on getting our health and nutritional priorities in order as a community. She wanted to talk to me because she was concerned about her daughter, Nicole, whose weight problems she had been ignoring for a long time. Nicole had been large at birth, Michelle told me, weighing in at 11 pounds, and she had remained large, but family members and friends had always just thought of her as "healthy." By age 8 she wore a size 16, but as Michelle explained, "Nobody bothered to keep track of her weight; we just knew she was getting to be too big for her age." Nicole had complained of kids teasing and taunting her at school, but Michelle and the family reassured her that she was loved at home and that there was really nothing to fret about.

But after hearing my speech, Michelle realized that because she and her husband were both heavyset and shared a family history of diabetes and cancer, she might be putting her daughter at risk by letting her remain so heavy. The fact that Michelle had already lost her youngest sister to breast cancer made her all the more determined to do something about her daughter's weight. She wasn't willing to lose her daughter to any disease that might be related to obesity.

With encouragement from me, Michelle decided to make some changes in her daughter's life. The first priority was to get Nicole moving, since she was, like so many overweight children, almost completely sedentary. So Michelle enrolled Nicole in a neighborhood soccer league and a local modern dance class. Next she knew she needed to change the whole family's eating habits. Michelle's family had been living on a steady diet of fast foods and other restaurant fare to save time in her and her husband's busy schedules. But her newly found commitment to health convinced her that it was important to keep ample fresh fruit and vegetables on hand for snacks and to reduce their fast-food fare to a once-a-month exception. Michelle says that before they made the changes there were times when their entire vegetable intake consisted of ketchup and french fries.

As Nicole's activities changed, so did her body. Today, a 9-year-old Nicole wears a size 10 and weighs 69 pounds, a noticeable difference from a year ago, and one that friends and classmates have been quick to applaud. She's a much happier child, too. At first she balked at the prospect of taking dance lessons, but now she can't wait to get there on Saturdays. And she loves her soccer game and the bicycle rides the family takes every weekend. Michelle says her greatest joy is when Nichole asks for an apple or for carrot sticks as snacks, rather than the chips, soda, and other high-fat, sugar-laden preferences of her past. "I know my baby has a fighting chance at being healthy, and because we've made changes with her, our whole family now has that same chance, too."

The Role of Obesity in Early-Onset Puberty

Another problem associated with overweight and obese children is early-onset puberty. In recent years, the number of elementary-school girls who look like high-schoolers and middle-school girls who look like they attend the local college has grown. Pediatricians nationwide are seeing girls 5 to 10 years old with breasts and pubic hair in alarming numbers—one out of seven white girls and an astonishing one out of every two African Americans. Though the reasons for this phenomenon are still being researched, experts see possible links to obesity, to the pesticides sprayed on fruits and veggies, and to hormones in beef and in cow's milk.

The link to weight seems a strong one, although it is not yet well understood. We have known for a while that very overweight girls start maturing earlier than their thinner peers, and it now appears that mildly overweight girls may be experiencing this early matu-ration as well. Dr. Paul Kaplowitz, a pediatric endocri-nologist at the Virginia Commonwealth University

School of Medicine, believes that the link between obesity and early maturation may be related to the hormone leptin. Since fat cells produce leptin, and since leptin is necessary for the progression of puberty, he believes the overweight and obesity epidemic may help to account for the growing numbers of preteen girls showing signs of early breast development. Another possible link between obesity and early puberty: Overweight girls have more insulin circulating in their bloodstream, and higher levels of insulin appear to stimulate the production of sex hormones from the ovaries and the adrenal glands.

Early puberty is a burden that can make the normal developmental and social challenges of growing up even more difficult. Girls who are still little more than children have no idea how to respond to the kind of attention they receive when their bodies grow up before they do. Being a child in a woman's body can cause acute psychological problems, including depression. Sistas, I don't have to tell you the havoc depression can wreak on our lives—and we're adults. Depressed children tend to become loners, spending more sedentary time in front of the TV or playing video games. It becomes a vicious cycle. So do your children a favor and help them change their lives.

Ignorance Is *Not* Bliss

For some reason, many people, including and especially African Americans, have missed or ignored the news about the dangers of overweight and obesity, tending instead to equate a fat child with a healthy child. The blinders don't get removed from our eyes as the child grows up, either. Excess padding tends to be more tolerated in the black community at any age. I know of a little boy who just celebrated his second birthday wearing clothing that would fit most 5-year-olds. His parents haven't been able to find a car seat that he can fit into comfortably. Though both parents are overweight (the mother's trying to slim down; the father isn't), they see nothing wrong with their gargantuan child. In fact, family members praise his size, believing it to be a sign that there's a football career in his future. His 6-year-old sister, by the way, is also on her way to heart attack city, weighing in at nearly 90 pounds. Both children eat all day long while parked in front of their DVD player, and you know they're not munching on apples, oranges, carrot sticks, and celery!

Baby Fat

You've probably heard that if a child is heavy during her toddler and preadolescent years, it's "just baby fat," a kind of weight gain that goes with being a child, right? You might have recognized this theory at work in Nicole's story above, in her family's response (or lack of response) to her weight. Well, unfortunately, there is no such thing, scientifically speaking, as baby fat, and a child who is overweight has the same predisposition for health problems that you do.

Monique's Story: ✦ Monique is a 14-year-old girl who stands five feet five inches, weighs 170 pounds, and was diagnosed with type II diabetes a year ago. Monique was the quintessential round baby, and

though she continued to be chubby all the way to adolescence, her parents, Deirdre and Andre, weren't worried because they thought it was just "baby fat" that
would somehow go away as she got older. But it didn't.
And her weight eventually ensured that she would develop diabetes—just like her mom, Deirdre, a faithful
Heart & Soul TV fan and frequent reader of the magazine, who has high blood pressure as well as diabetes.
Although she and her husband had long since accepted their own weight problems, Deirdre was hor-
rified when she discovered that her baby girl had
developed the same disease that had made her own
life so difficult.

Monique's diabetes forced Deirdre to take a long,
hard look at her family's way of life. In an effort to save
her daughter's health and spare her from years of hu-
miliation, she decided to do something about the way
they had been living. Today, Monique does not take
part in any organized sports, but she walks for an hour
four times a week with her mom and dad. That part
she found fun. The idea of changing her diet, however,
was not. But the combination of the cruelty of her
peers, who ragged her constantly about her weight,
and a talk with her mom and her endocrinologist
about what diabetes would do to her convinced her to
try. Her first change was cutting out sweets, her "best
friend" for the past decade. Monique admits to having
had a "chocolate addiction." At her mother's sugges-
tion, after tackling sweets she next agreed to replace
the sodas she had made a part of her daily diet with
water and some juice. Deirdre has worked very hard to
help Monique, using suggestions from me that have

resulted in a weight loss of 40 pounds. The hard part of Monique's weight battle isn't over, however, because not only does she have another 20 or 30 pounds to go, but then she'll have to face the challenge of keeping those pounds off. My guess is she'll succeed. With her mother's help she has managed to craft a healthy eating plan for herself by keeping away from foods that she has learned sabotage her—fats, sweets, and high-calorie junk foods. And she loves the fact that so many people notice her new look. For now, she's happy with how far she has come, and determined to stay the course. Bravo!

It's Never Too Early for Veggies

If you're thinking that it's silly to focus so much attention on nutrition for your perfectly healthy, happy kids, consider these facts: More than 84 percent of children consume too much total fat, and more than 91 percent consume too much saturated fat—the kind of fat in meat and dairy products. Conversely, 91 percent of children between the ages of 6 and 11 *don't* eat the recommended minimum of five servings of fruits and vegetables a day. Clearly, children are not at fault for these ridiculous numbers. The blame lies squarely at your parental feet. Yes, I know it's easier to get them to eat french fries than spinach, but that's probably because they were offered french fries long before they ever saw fresh-cooked spinach.

All babies are born with taste buds that have a preference for sweet things, while their taste for other flavors must be developed. This is why as a nutritionist, I encourage parents to introduce infants to puréed vegetables as soon as they're ready to progress beyond milk and cereals, even before fruits. Otherwise the child will learn to prefer the sweet taste of the fruit and will be much less willing to try the vegetables. As the child gets older, repeated and early introductions to such healthy fare as vegetables, whole grains, dried beans, and other healthy foods can help you win the battle against the fast-food chains. While you're trying to mold your child's food preferences, remember that kids often dislike vegetables with a certain texture and mouth feel; think gritty lima beans or slimy okra. All this means is that you must make your vegetable choices carefully, opting for those that are more likely to appeal to them. You should also try to prepare vegetables in an appetizing way: For example, steam green beans and lightly stir-fry other veggies, rather than cooking them to a slow death. And if you're the mom who promises a piece of candy or cake as a reward for eating carrots, this can backfire. You don't want to use dessert to bribe kids into eating nutritious food. If Ray-Ray is given one food as a reward, he will learn to prefer that food, and his vegetables will probably be tossed in the dog's bowl. The truth is, if you oven-roast your carrots until they are slightly brown and caramelized on the outside, they'll be so sweet and appetizing that they'll have just as much appeal to your child's taste buds as the cake—so no reward for eating them will be needed.

Tips for Tots

So what else can you do to ensure that your children get the recommended daily amount of vitamins and minerals and the wide variety of nutrients they need to grow, thrive, and stay healthy? How can you convince children who love potato chips that spinach is just as yummy? Here are some tips to help make healthy food seem like an attractive alternative to junk food:

❖ Limit the amount of junk food, including soda and juice drinks, in your home. Children can't eat food you don't have. Don't buy the stuff and then pronounce it off-limits—this only makes forbidden foods seem all the more desirable. So keep your purchases of junk food to a minimum.

❖ Set a good example. Many children follow their parents' lead when it comes to eating. If you follow healthy and nutritious eating patterns, it's likely your children will, too.

❖ Offer your children lots of options. Many children are still developing a taste for food. Just because they don't like one vegetable doesn't mean they won't like others. Try offering them a variety of healthy foods. And don't give up—even though you were able to entice Ray-Ray to eat those roasted carrots and Maddy has no use for them, that doesn't mean she's a lost cause. Like adults, children have different palates. But every child can learn to like at least a few vegetables and fruits.

❖ For toddlers, cut foods into unusual and creative shapes. Making food fun sometimes makes it more enticing, especially for younger children.

❖ Put food into fun containers. Preparing a meal and storing it in individual containers allows you to control portion size. And using fun containers or applying decals or stickers makes mealtime more festive.

❖ Have your child participate in meal preparation. Children who are able to participate and help select the ingredients when preparing meals may be more receptive to eating the finished product.

❖ Plant a vegetable garden. Let your child help tend a home-grown vegetable patch. He or she may be proud to enjoy the bounty of your joint labors.

❖ Prepare foods in unusual ways. Why don't you stick a tomato in the blender and let your child drink the result? Have fun, and be creative!

Getting Heart-Smart About Protecting Your Greatest Asset

Since science has already taught us that kids with high cholesterol become adults with the same problem (this is almost guaranteed if they're overweight), you must take precautions to protect them against this and other risk factors for heart disease. Besides the cholesterol risk factor, it should also be noted that children with high blood pressure are likely to become adults with high blood pressure if the condition is left unchecked. If your child was born into a family with a history of high cholesterol or heart disease, you should have your child's cholesterol checked as early as age 2.

Pediatricians agree that if the child's total cholesterol is 170 mg/dl or higher and the LDL (bad) cholesterol is 110 mg/dl or higher, you need to pay close attention to his diet, selecting foods that will protect your child from becoming one more addition to the pool of heart disease statistics for black folks. Start your child's heart-healthy program by making the right food choices.

You should also think about stepping up your child's physical activity. That means get that child movin'!

Healthy Snack Suggestions for Children

Whole grain cereals
Cheese
Cheese sticks
Whole-grain crackers
Dried fruits (children
    younger than 3 should
    not eat dried fruit
    because it can be a
    choking hazard; it also
    promotes cavities)
Fresh fruits
Fresh vegetables
Hard-boiled eggs
Whole-grain muffins
Peanut butter
Popcorn
Sugar-free pudding
Sherbet
Broth-based soups made
    with vegetables
Tuna

Start Your Child's Engine Early

It's never too early to put your child on the road to an active lifestyle. Many youngsters spend too much time confined to strollers, swings, baby seats, and playpens. This is usually because we want to keep our children safe while we get things done. Instead of "containerizing" our babies, however, we should learn to let them out—in a safe environment, of course—to move.

Now, I'm not suggesting a full-fledged aerobic workout for babies. I'm talking about fun activities that make being physical a normal part of everyday life in the hope that children will not grow up to be among the 60 percent of us who are overweight couch potatoes.

Parents usually assume that skills such as rolling over, sitting up, and walking will just come naturally as babies grow. According to pediatric specialists, however, babies need the right environment to connect the brain to the muscles that perform these activities. For example, an infant who spends a large part of the day in a bouncy seat may like watching the suspended toys, but he or she will probably roll over or sit up later than babies who spend more time stretching out on a blanket.

Though it may seem to you that your young children move around a lot, they aren't always getting all the physical activity they need. TV and video games keep large numbers of preschoolers sedentary for longer than parents may realize. And for older children there are far too few playgrounds where parents can feel secure about allowing their children to play unsupervised.

All children need opportunities to be physically active, but different activities are needed at different ages to spark development. Keep the following tips in mind:

❖ Part of an infant's day should be spent in structured activity with a parent or caregiver—playing peek-aboo or patty-cake, being carried to and exploring new environments.

❖ Do not keep infants or toddlers in baby seats or other restrictive settings for long periods. Even young infants move differently when placed on a blanket on the floor than when in a baby seat.

❖ Toddlers should have at least 30 minutes of structured physical activity and preschoolers at least an hour during each day. Play follow-along songs, chase, or ball. For older children, balancing games and tumbling increase strength and body control.

❖ Toddlers and preschoolers should spend at least an hour, preferably more, a day in free play—exploring, experimenting, imitating. Caregivers should provide safe objects to ride, push, pull, balance on, and climb.

❖ Toddlers and preschoolers should not be sedentary for more than an hour at a time, except when they are sleeping.

❖ Bring along your friend's children for playtime. Research shows that children who are alone a lot are more likely to lead sedentary lifestyles.

❖ Don't force physical activity or use it as punishment. Instead, it should be a routine part of daily life, and you should join in, not just sit on a park bench and watch the children romp. By all means, make it fun.

Heart-Healthy Foods for Children

Baked chicken nuggets (made of skinless chicken breast)

Reduced-fat mac and cheese (made of reduced-fat cheddar, fat-free or reduced-fat milk, and frozen veggies)

Whole-wheat tortillas filled with lean chicken strips and topped with vegetables

Fruit-berry sorbet in a wafer cone

Milk shakes (made with low-fat frozen yogurt and a small sandwich cookie)

Homemade pizza (made of whole-grain English muffins, reduced-fat cheese, and lots of veggies)

Soy fruit shakes

Fruit roll-ups

Helping Your Sedentary Older Children to Get Movin'

So you didn't get your child active when she was a toddler; it's never too late to start. In addition to helping to reduce the risk of obesity-related illnesses, physical activity helps increase a child's alertness and attention span, which can lead to better academic performance.

For starters, peel your child away from the TV. Experts recommend limiting their TV-watching time to no more than an hour per day; one study of third and fourth graders who were only allowed to watch one hour of TV a day found they had lost considerable weight in a nine-month period. Then encourage your child to get involved in a team sport. For many children, team sports such as baseball, soccer, and basketball enable them to stay physically active on a regular basis and will also plug them into a social network—a good deterrent to hiding away by themselves in their rooms, lost in a TV show or a computer game.

Ashaad's Story: ✦ Ten-year-old Ashaad is a perfect example of the benefits of team sports. According to Cheryl and Roscoe, Ashaad's parents, he had gradually put on a great deal of weight during a three-year period when Roscoe was sick and no longer able to participate in father-son sports activities with Ashaad or to take him to karate classes as he had previously done. Worried about his father's illness, and with fewer outlets for being active, Ashaad began to spend all his spare time in front of the television set and the computer. By the time he was 8, and before his mom was even aware of what was happening, Ashaad had gained 60 pounds! "I was floored when his pediatrician announced his weight," Cheryl recalled. The issue of his weight really came to a head because he wanted to play on a football team at school. But at 8, he was supposed to play on the team for 75-pound boys. Weighing in at 142 pounds, he didn't have a prayer of being able to play on that team, or even on the team for 12-year-old boys weighing 85 and under. So the coach sent him packing.

"He was so disappointed, and we were at a loss for how to comfort him. That was when we knew we had to do something to help our son," Roscoe explained. With a family history of heart disease on his father's side and of obesity on his mother's, there was more than football at stake for Ashaad. And there was also Ashaad's younger sister, 5-year-old Akeyla, to consider. She would be inheriting the same family legacy of disease risks if the family didn't make changes in their lifestyle, Cheryl and Roscoe realized.

So they began to ease into a new way of life, beginning with a whole new approach to breakfast. They started the day with oatmeal and fruit. "We thought if we could replace the bacon-and-egg breakfasts with something more healthy, we might be off to a good start." They were. The kids accepted their new menus without much fuss, and gradually they accepted the changes Cheryl made in their other meals as well. Next Roscoe enrolled Ashaad in basketball and soccer tournaments to get him moving and improve his cardiovascular health. "Since my mother had heart disease," he explained, "we worried that Ashaad might have inherited some things from his grandma that we wouldn't want him to get. It took a while, but we've finally got Ashaad's weight almost back to a normal range. What happened to him taught us to pull together as a family to take care of ourselves." The kids now ride bikes with their mom in a nearby park. They also Rollerblade, ride scooters, and go out to the local playground to play with their friends almost every day. Best of all, Ashaad is now on two teams—basketball and football. "He's much happier now, and we worry less about his health," says a very proud Cheryl.

Before your child takes to the field, you should consider a few things. First, be sure the child gets a physical exam before playing any challenging competitive sport, so that you'll be confident there are no conditions that would preclude participation. Second, if he or she has spent the summer as a couch potato or lacks physical conditioning, tell the coach; coaches should develop training programs for their players that are tailored to age as well as physical abilities.

However, don't force your child to participate in a sport if he or she really doesn't like that sport. You can help keep children in shape by encouraging them to participate in all kinds of activities that don't involve sports—raking leaves, bicycling, ice-skating, Rollerblading, walking for a cause, weight lifting, or something as simple but physically rewarding as washing the car.

A special note about teen girls: According to a recent study, which followed 1,213 black girls and 1,166 white girls from the Washington, D.C., Cincinnati, and San Francisco areas for 10 years, the amount of regular exercise girls get falls off dramatically as they move through their teenage years, dropping to practically zero in many cases, and among black girls in particular. In fact, by the time they were 16 or 17, more than half of the black girls in the study said they got no regular

Get Your Kids Walking to School

Only a quarter of the children in this country walk or bicycle to school, which may be a contributing factor to the country's growing problem of childhood obesity. Apparently, just as adults roll out of bed and into the car to drive to work, the children are also in tow—being driven to school by their parents, or riding on the school bus or public transportation. According to the CDC's study, the first national one of its kind, distance, weather, traffic, and crime are the main reasons parents cite for not allowing or encouraging their children to walk to school.

In some communities, however, parents are fighting back against crime and other safety hazards in an effort to keep their kids active. In one California community, a two-year campaign for safer walking paths and bike lanes doubled the number of students who used them. In another, the parent-teacher organization asked parents to walk their kids' routes to school and keep a list of hazards, such as uneven sidewalks or intersections without crosswalks. Then the parents lobbied the local government to fix the problems. The number of children walking has nearly doubled in that community as well. Even without such community strength, many parents have realized they can organize on a smaller level by joining with several other parents and organizing a sort of "walk pool," in which groups of children walk to and from school together as protection against potential attackers. Safety in numbers is always a good idea.

exercise at all outside school. The study found that the decline of physical activity among girls was affected by lower levels of parental education, heavier weight, smoking, and pregnancy. Though no similar study of teenage boys' physical activity has been done, the study's authors say boys tend to be more active because of their greater participation in team sports.

Another significant finding of this study is that obesity rates among the girls doubled, even though no significant increase in caloric consumption was reported. Makes you put that index finger to the side of your temple and go "hmmm." You'd have to admit, that's a pretty strong case for the value of getting a move on.

Be a Role Model

Children whose parents are active are six times more likely to be active than children whose parents are couch potatoes. Conversely, obese parents tend to have obese children. In fact, if you and your child's father are obese, your child is 80 percent more likely to tip the scales on the extremely heavy side. So step out there with your child. In addition to setting an example for your child about maintaining an active lifestyle, you'll be able to spend quality time together as a family.

Checklist for Jump-Starting Your Children

Sure, you know that it's important for your children to get exercise, and you keep telling them to go out and play. But they don't, and you quietly give in to their TV and/or computer addiction. Before caving so easily, ask yourself the following questions:

- ❧ How much time do my children spend sitting in front of the television or in front of the computer? And how does that compare to the amount of time I spend being sedentary?
- ❧ What kind of space is there in my yard for play? Are there adequate play areas near my home?
- ❧ Have I provided them with the resources to be active—a bike, a basketball hoop, an area in the yard to kick a ball around?
- ❧ Is there a walking path near my home? Or can they walk around the block a few times?
- ❧ Are there running or walking tracks nearby?
- ❧ What type of physical education program, if any, does my children's school offer? What can I do to increase physical education class offerings at my child's school?
- ❧ Do we engage in physical activities as a family?
- ❧ What kinds of physical activities do my kids enjoy doing? Have I done everything I could to encourage them?
- ❧ Is my child overweight, or does my child have any physical illness or limitation—and what is the pediatrician's advice on exercise?
- ❧ Have I provided support and encouragement for physical pursuits?
- ❧ Have I provided a role model for physical fitness?

If your answers say you haven't done the things necessary to get your children on the right track for a healthy, normal-weight lifestyle, you've got to make things right. So throw out the fatback, dust off your vegetable steamer, and make a walking date for your family. Use the nutrition and fitness information in this book and start a Dr. Ro Livin' Healthy Club (see Secret 10) with your family and friends. You could even start one at your church and extend it to your entire community!

Raising Strong Girls

In a book about living healthy for African American women, I would be remiss if I ignored our precious jewels, our young girls. So much is written about the plight of young black males, and it is true that our sons are endangered in ways no other group of young people is. But young sistas also face many challenges in today's society: doing well in school, fitting in with peers, finding their place in the world. They also face some serious social challenges—sexual pressures, drugs, pregnancy, sexually transmitted diseases, physical and verbal abuse—that can alter the very course of their lives. Many of these issues are even harder to confront for girls with low self-esteem, and that's why I'm talking about self-esteem in a book about nutrition, because an overweight, out-of-shape girl already has several strikes against her in the self-esteem department. A black girl is likely to have several more.

Fostering a healthy sense of self is one of the most important jobs for parents who are raising African

American girls. For our daughters, the foundation for that strong sense of self is a nurturing and supportive family life. How can you make sure you're doing enough to nurture your daughter's self-esteem? The most important thing is communication. Talk to your daughter. Ask her what's going on in school and with her peers. Talk about television, music, and magazines; girls are exposed to many images from these media, from scantily clad dancers in music videos to stick-thin models in magazines, that can negatively affect how they see themselves. The strong anti-female bias of a lot of hip-hop and rap lyrics may further undermine their feelings about themselves. And even though some studies have suggested that black girls tend to have stronger body images than white girls, our daughters are far from immune to the insidious messages out there.

Girls often worry about their physical attractiveness, and many aspects of our society do not validate black girls' looks. Even within our own community we're still struggling with stereotypes about skin tone and hair texture. You still hear black people say, "She has good hair," referring to softly wavy or straight hair. And you also hear, "She's pretty for a dark-skinned girl." As a young girl of a darker hue, I faced this kind of prejudice myself when I was growing up. I face it now as an adult, too. Pop culture still tends to put a higher value on black women with fairer complexions, as any look at the biggest movie stars and most successful musicians will bear out. Because of such preferences, we have to be vigilant about reminding our black daughters about the wonderful diversity of hues that characterizes our race.

Positive parenting can do much to offset the influences within mainstream media and our own culture. My own mother, Larvenia, was a dark-skinned woman whose family was much the same. On the other hand, my guardian was a fair-skinned woman from a long line of fair-skinned people. But both of them made sure to let me know I was someone very special, because they knew about the prejudice that was "waiting out there for her," as I heard my mother say many times when she didn't think I was listening. This was one of the most important things either of my mamas could have done for me, and they did it constantly, day in, day out. Every day I heard "I love you," "You are so pretty," "How beautiful you look today." You can do the same for your daughters. Here is some practical advice to help keep their sense of self strong:

✤ Encourage your daughter to value her own beauty, whatever form it takes. Be proactive in setting and communicating your own standards of beauty—inner and outer—and your daughter will learn to appreciate the uniqueness of each person's beauty, including her own.

✤ Help your daughter appreciate her own accomplishments. The diverse achievements of black women have not always been recognized. They may not get the recognition for their achievements immediately, but that doesn't mean they did not achieve.

✤ Reassure your daughter she does not have to fit into the stereotyped portrayals of black women seen on television and in movies. On TV, the black girls who seem meek are the ones who get all the approval. Those on-screen images send black girls the message that you will be accepted only if you're not too confident or too assertive. If you stand up for yourself, chances are you will be seen as aggressive.

❖ Support your daughter's development and exploration of her own character and opinions. Black girls should be encouraged to place a high value on being accepted and respected for their individual qualities, and they should not feel that they need to apologize for their strengths. They must also know that their worth and self-concept must be determined by them, not by anyone else.

❖ Teach your daughter that it is not okay for women to be disrespected. Encourage her to refuse to accept any kind of abuse, physical or verbal. Every black girl should believe she deserves better than that. If we don't teach our daughters this, we've failed them.

❖ Help your daughter develop a positive attitude about her body. Although young girls are often mortified at being teased about their developing breasts, they should embrace those changes as part of womanhood.

❖ Make sure your daughter knows that she has a right—and a responsibility—to define what is acceptable behavior and to set limits. All girls should understand that it is okay to speak out if someone else's behavior makes them uncomfortable. If a boy has written a letter or makes comments to your daughter that are out of line, help her stand up for herself. Let her know she has to be all right with her body and personal space. Help her to recognize inappropriate behavior and to understand how to respond.

A Poem About Self-Image
"Good Hair"
by Dr. Ro

Sick and tired of your tresses?
Always a mess
Genetics gave you a raw deal
'Cause your hair's not the best

So you blow-dry and perm it
And straighten till dawn
Turn the hot comb on high
And press right on

Didn't think hair could make you
So confused till this day
Always a-frettin' and a-primpin'
To get it just the right way

Baby's daddy's is curly
To make it good for the next
Generation to love him
He'll pass the hair test

A WOMAN'S CRO-W-N IS HER GLORY!
Your mama's words ring out
What a sad thing to ponder
And still judge people by

The truth about hair?
Whether black, brown, or red
Only thing good about it
Is that it's ON YOUR HEAD

Frequently Asked Questions

Q Dr. Ro: My 10-year-old-daughter is over-weight. I've tried everything from locking the cabinets to punishing her for stealing food. I no longer buy snack food, and I pack only healthy things in her lunch. Still, she manages to get her hands on candy bars and fast food at every turn. Getting her to be physically active has also been a problem; she is so heavy it is difficult for her to partic-ipate, and during team sports she's usually the last person picked to play. I can't afford one of those fat-kid camps I keep hearing about on the news. Help!

A *Cajoling, punishing, and berating your daughter won't get her to stop eating junk and fast food on the sly. Indeed, it might have the oppo-site effect: The more you threaten, the more likely she will find ways to circumvent your threats. And even if you could afford a summer camp for children with weight issues, it wouldn't work in the long run unless your daughter's entire lifestyle changes. Otherwise, she would probably take off weight during the camp, then put it back on, plus some, when she returns home.*

My best advice is to keep lots of low-calorie, nutritious food in the house and encourage her to eat it when she's hungry and to stop when she's full. Don't wait for her to get her physical activity at school, especially since she doesn't excel at team sports; instead, go on long walks with her. Better yet, start the whole family on a walking regimen. You mentioned that you no longer buy junk food, and you pack healthy lunches for your daughter. Are you preparing healthy meals at other times? And is the whole family eating more fruits and vegetables and fewer fatty foods? Because if not, she's likely to feel singled out and victimized by being made to eat different foods from the rest of you. Make healthy eating a family affair.

Then—and this will probably be the hardest part— let go. Once you've done everything you can, don't comment on her weight. She may need time to make her own commitment to change, without pressure from you. If things don't get better, you may need to take your daughter to see her pediatrician for other suggestions on how you—and she—can get her weight under control.

Q Dr. Ro: We have made nutritional changes at my house, limiting fatty junk food and increasing fruits, vegetables, and whole grains. But my mother keeps my children for about three hours after school each day, and I can't convince her not to give the kids junk. Even when I take food to her house for her to feed them, she insists on giving them candy, cake, and cookies, saying, "There's nothing wrong with children having something a little sweet now and then." The problem is, it's not now and then. Having someone else watch the kids is not an option. What can I do?

A *First, kudos to you for making the changes necessary to keep your family healthy! Your children seem to be adjusting to the changes, but your mother is a different story. Unlike a child-care provider who isn't a family member, your mother probably won't respond to demands that she stop doling out fatty, sugarladen snacks. You can, however, explain the benefits of healthy nutrition. Tell her you are trying to keep the children from inheriting the legacy of diabetes, high blood pressure, cancer, and heart disease prevalent in so many black families. I know from personal experience how difficult it is to teach old dogs new tricks, so you'll have to be persistent yet patient with her.*

Try a compromise: Tell her that you are okay with the children having one cookie apiece, in addition to whatever healthy foodstuffs you've packed for them, but several cookies and big hunks of cake on a regular basis are out. Another thought: If you are packing after-school snacks for the kids to eat and they are eating those snacks, perhaps they will be too full to eat much of the sweet stuff their grandmother insists on providing for them.

Q Dr. Ro: Isn't all this focus on diet and exercise going to give my daughter an eating disorder?

A If you give your children an early start on a healthy lifestyle, eating nutritious foods and being active will seem like a natural part of life, not a "focus on diet and exercise." That said, you should know that studies show that black girls tend to have better self-images than their white counterparts, which may be why they don't suffer eating disorders as often as white girls, since eating disorders like anorexia nervosa and bulimia involve self-critical, negative thoughts and feelings about appearance.

Eating disorders consist of eating behaviors so extreme that they harm normal body composition and functioning. A person with anorexia nervosa typically starves herself to be thin. Bulimia is characterized by binge eating and purging. Both disorders may also be characterized by compulsive exercise.

Your behavior as a parent may help your child to avoid eating disorders. Encourage, don't belittle, your child daily. Focus on your child's strengths, and you will build self-esteem. Base your child's self-esteem on who she is and what she does, not how much she weighs. Work on making a healthy body the ideal of beauty. And remember, your own body image may influence your child's body image. If she hears you constantly *complaining about how fat you are and watches you starting and stopping diets all the time, your daughter may feel that it is normal and acceptable to have a distorted relationship to food and a poor body image.*

Finally, illustrate what a healthy lifestyle is to your child. Involve your child in the preparation of healthy, nutritious meals. Let her know that it's okay to eat when you're hungry and refuse food when you're not. Also, make exercise a fun and rewarding family activity, as well as a regular one. If you have healthy attitudes about food and exercise, your child will have a good example from which to learn.

Q **Dr. Ro: My son isn't overweight, but I'd like to get him more physically active just for the health benefits. But he's not athletically inclined at all; actually, he's a little on the clumsy side. What can we do besides walking?**

A *If your son can't navigate a bicycle or Rollerblades, and joining the football team is out of the question, try something a little less likely to cause an injury. Toss a Frisbee, where the point isn't his athletic ability but having fun. Encourage your son to try his hand at martial arts, horseback riding, swimming, or hiking. As long as your son does not become sedentary, there's no reason to worry if he resists joining organized sports activities.*

Q   Dr. Ro: My 3-year-old child is a picky eater, and I don't know what to do. Also, do I need to give her a multivitamin?

A   *I feel your pain—one day your daughter can't get enough bananas, the next day she throws a temper tantrum and swears she's never liked them. It's a familiar challenge. Don't let this discourage you from continuing to put these foods in front of her. Monitor the amount of liquid she drinks; she could be too full to eat her food. Try not to let her have more than 20 to 30 ounces of liquid—milk, juice, water—each day, and don't let her drink within an hour before meals or while she is eating her meal.*

If you still have difficulty getting your picky eater to eat enough fruits and veggies, a chewable multivitamin will help. Don't let her have a brand that gives her more than 100 percent of the recommended daily allowance of any one vitamin or mineral. Also make sure the vitamin you choose has iron in it. Vitamins are not a cure-all, but they will help until your daughter is through this phase.

Secret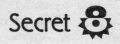

To Supplement or Not to Supplement: That Is the Question

 In this insta-world, we have come to expect instant gratification. I'm sure you know people who want the weight off yesterday. How many times have you heard "I have to lose 10 pounds by next Friday so I can fit into a size 6 dress for cousin Brenda's wedding"? So when instant gratification becomes the rule of the day, healing in a pill is the desired cure-all for good health. Although this is unrealistic, there *are* some supplements that can improve your health and may help in your quest to prevent disease, as long as you keep in mind that they are *only* supplements to a good diet, not replacements for one.

The Dietary Supplement Health and Education Act defines dietary supplements as products (other than tobacco) that contain a vitamin, mineral, amino acid, herb, and/or other botanical and are intended to supplement a person's diet. Dietary supplements are available widely through many commercial sources, including health food and grocery stores, pharmacies, and mail-order suppliers. They come in many forms, from tablets and capsules to powders, gel-tabs, extracts, and liquids. In the past, the most common type of dietary supplement in this country was a multivitamin/mineral tablet or capsule. Supplements containing strictly herbal preparations were less widely known and used. Now a wide variety of supplement products is available, and some include vitamins, minerals, other nutrients, and various herbal and botanical supplements, as well as ingredients and extracts of animal origin.

Your body needs vitamins and minerals in small amounts for normal growth, function, and health. But your body doesn't make most of the vitamins and minerals it needs, so you must get these micronutrients from the fluids you drink, the plants and animal products you eat, or in some cases from supplements.

Vitamins

You need vitamins for normal body function, mental alertness, and resistance to infection. They enable your body to process proteins, carbohydrates, and fats. Certain vitamins also help produce blood cells, hormones, genetic material, and chemicals in your nervous system. There are 14 vitamins, which fall into two categories:

❖ *Fat-soluble*. Vitamins A, D, E, and K. They're stored in your body's fat. Some fat-soluble vitamins, such as vitamins A and D, can accumulate in your body and reach toxic levels.

❖ *Water-soluble.* Vitamin C, choline, biotin, and the seven B vitamins: thiamin (B_1), riboflavin (B_2), niacin (B_3), pantothenic acid (B_5), pyridoxine (B_6), folic acid/folate (B_9), and cobalamin (B_{12}). They're stored to a lesser extent than fat-soluble vitamins.

Minerals

Recently I read a health newsletter that compared the human body to a sturdy building, because both rely on minerals for much of their strength, and both are built to last. That really captures what minerals do for you. Major minerals—those your body needs in larger amounts—include calcium, phosphorus, magnesium, sodium, potassium, and chloride. Calcium, phosphorus, and magnesium are important in the development and health of your bones and teeth. Sodium, potassium, and chloride, known as electrolytes, are important in regulating the water and chemical balance in your body. In addition, your body needs smaller amounts of what are known as the trace minerals—chromium, copper, fluoride, iodine, iron, manganese, molybdenum, selenium, and zinc. Together with the major minerals, they play crucial roles in numerous body functions and are found in every fluid, tissue, cell, and organ.

Finding the Balance

Having the right balance of vitamins and minerals in your body is essential, because prolonged vitamin or mineral deficiencies can cause specific diseases or conditions, such as night blindness (vitamin A deficiency), pernicious anemia (vitamin B_{12} deficiency), or iron deficiency anemia.

So are these herbal and vitamin concoctions magic bullets that will make us well? Hardly. In fact, some experts say you should take the latest developments in the supplement world with a healthy dose of skepticism. But with what now adds up to a $6 billion dietary supplement industry, America has bought the bill of goods some folks are selling. Most people think it's possible to eat whatever they want, take a vitamin or some form of herbal supplement, and go happily on their way to the land of the healthy and free.

African Americans are no exception. We want to heal ourselves, too. And we want to do it as quickly, as effortlessly, and as painlessly as humanly possible.

Veggies in a Pill

Looking over the latest offerings in the nutrition arena, you may not be surprised to see that some companies actually claim to have figured out how to "capsulate" what you need from vegetables into a pill. I'm not talking about the requisite multivitamin that you've been told to pop each day. No siree, these are vegetables crammed into pills. That's right, they're literally veggie pills.

Should you get your vegetables in a pill to prevent disease? Here's what the science says: Keep eating your vegetables just like your grandma has been preaching for as long as you can remember, because taking a pill isn't good enough. Although some brands claim that each tablet or capsule contains a serving of vegetables, it's practically impossible to fit the nutritional value of a serving of vegetables into a capsule. Furthermore, no research to date has proven that taking vegetables in concentrated pill form gives the same protection from disease that you would get from the actual foods that contain the disease-fighting phytochemicals and antioxidants. The process of dehydrating and concentrating the vegetables to put them in this form damages the nutrition offered by the veggies in the first place. So much of the vitamin content is likely to be leached out during the processing that even Shaft on his best day wouldn't be able to find the nutrient.

To get an idea of what one of these pills actually offers, let's look at the label for Nature's Plus Mixed Vegetables brand, which boasts that each capsule contains about 10,000 milligrams of fresh broccoli and 1,000 milligrams each of spinach, cabbage, and carrots. But once you consider that you'd have to take four and a half capsules to get the vitamins A and C and the folate found in a single serving of broccoli, it doesn't sound so inviting anymore. To get the vitamins A and C found in a serving of spinach, think about taking 56, count 'em, 56 capsules. Or 70 capsules to get the equivalent of the vitamins A and C and the mineral phosphorus found in a serving of raw cabbage. And wouldn't you really rather eat one medium carrot to get the vitamin A and beta-carotene it provides instead of taking 72 capsules? When it comes to the veggie pill option, I'd have to say thanks just the same, but I'd rather get my vegetables from the produce section.

Is There Energy in Vitamins?

In my more than two decades as a practicing nutritionist I've heard too many folks claim that they take vitamins for energy. If I've heard this once, I've heard it a thousand times. As a nutritionist, I am the first to agree that we should all take at least a multivitamin/mineral daily. Do I recommend that you do so for energy? Not a chance. Here's why: Vitamins do not supply energy. Carbohydrates and fat provide energy. Still, vitamins are essential because they assist the process of releasing energy from the foods you eat. Bottom line? Vitamins do not produce energy on their own, but they are a necessary factor in energy release.

Whole Foods Versus Dietary Supplements

No matter how helpful they may be, supplements can't save you from a bad diet! Despite the fact that food industry zealots have taken a nugget of truth and run with it, there is no proof that taking your nutrient in pill form will have the same helpful effects as eating daily servings of the food that contain them naturally.

For example, you can get your entire daily requirement of vitamin C by popping a pill. You can also get it by eating a large orange. So which is better? The orange, a whole food, is much better. In fact, whole foods—fruits, vegetables, grains, lean meats, and dairy products—have two main benefits you can't find in a pill.

First, whole foods are complex, containing a wide variety of the nutrients your body needs—including nutrients we have not yet identified but are sure to discover in years to come—so you get much more bang for your nutrition buck. Fruits and vegetables, for example, contain phytochemicals, which, as we have discussed, are naturally occurring substances that may help protect you against cancer, heart disease, osteoporosis, and diabetes. Take that orange we were just discussing: It provides vitamin C, but it also has beta-carotene, calcium, and other disease-fighting nutrients the supplement lacks. Similarly, you get not just bone-building calcium from a glass of milk but protein, vitamin D, riboflavin, calcium, phosphorus, and magnesium. But if you take only calcium supplements and skip calcium-rich foods, such as low-fat milk, yogurt, or calcium-fortified soy products, you may miss these other nutrients, a number of which you need for healthy bones.

Second, whole foods provide dietary fiber. Fiber is important for digestion and to help prevent certain diseases. It is also, as I mentioned in Secret 3, beneficial in keeping the weight off. Soluble fiber, found in certain beans and grains and in some fruits and vegetables, helps prevent heart disease by reducing cholesterol and helps prevent or control diabetes by regulating glucose levels in the blood. Insoluble fiber, found in whole grains and in some vegetables and fruits, helps move food through the intestines and thus helps to prevent constipation.

A Short Primer on Food Sources for Nutrients

Now that you understand how important it is to get most of your vitamins and minerals from whole food sources whenever possible, you'll want to know where to find them. Following is a list of the nutrients your body needs to function properly, and of the foods in which they can be found. You can go to Table 8-1 for information about what these nutrients actually do for you.

Vitamins

Biotin: ✦ Because your body needs only a small amount of biotin, some of which is produced by bacteria in your intestines, your diet usually supplies enough without your needing to get any more from a supplement. Rich sources of this vitamin are egg yolk, liver, and brewer's yeast. Although I have recommended using egg whites for a high-protein, low-fat alternative to whole eggs, I'm not anti-yolk. In fact, recent studies have exonerated egg yolks from the bad rap they received in the past. For a while, eating more than three a week was considered akin to committing one of the seven deadly sins, because they were thought to increase cholesterol levels. But a Harvard School of Public Health study found no relationship between egg consumption and cardiovascular disease. In a population of more than 117,000 nurses and health professionals that was followed for 8 to 14 years, there was no difference in heart disease rates between those who consumed less than one egg a week and those who ate more than one egg a day. Another factor in the anti-egg prejudice of the past was the salmonella scare of the mid-1980s. To combat the risk of salmonella, simply make sure you cook your eggs thoroughly before eating them.

Folic Acid (B9): ✦ Most bread in this country has added folic acid. Green leafy vegetables such as spinach, turnip greens, and mustard greens are rich sources of folate. Citrus fruit and juices, legumes, fortified cereals, and wheat germ are other excellent sources of folate.

Niacin (B3): ✦ Good sources for this B vitamin include brewer's yeast, meat, poultry, fish (tuna, salmon), cereals (especially fortified ones), legumes, and seeds. Milk, green leafy vegetables, coffee, and tea also provide some niacin.

Pantothenic Acid (B5): ✦ Liver, kidney, brewer's yeast, egg yolk, broccoli, fish, shellfish, chicken, milk, yogurt, legumes, mushrooms, avocados, and sweet potatoes are the best sources for this B vitamin. Whole grains are also good sources of pantothenic acid, but processing may result in a 35 to 75 percent loss in the vitamin's effectiveness. Freezing and canning foods cause similar losses.

Riboflavin (B$_2$): ✦ You can find riboflavin in fortified cereals, milk, cheddar cheese, almonds, asparagus, and chicken.

Thiamin (B$_1$): ✦ This vitamin can be found in whole-grain cereals, legumes, nuts, and brewer's yeast.

Vitamin B$_6$: ✦ Bananas, turkey, salmon, hazelnuts, spinach, and chicken are all relatively rich sources of vitamin B$_6$. People who follow a very restricted vegetarian diet might need to increase their B$_6$ intake by eating food fortified with this vitamin, like fortified cereals, or by taking a supplement.

Vitamin B$_{12}$: ✦ This vitamin is present only in animal products, including meat, poultry, fish (including shellfish), and to a lesser extent milk. People who follow vegan diets (no animal foods of any kind) need to obtain this vitamin in a supplement.

Vitamin A: ✦ Good sources of vitamin A include sweet potatoes, butternut squash, zucchini, cantaloupe, raw carrots, apricots, and spinach.

Vitamin C: ✦ Unlike most mammals, we humans don't have the ability to make our own vitamin C, so we have to get it through diet or supplements. Fortunately, there are many good whole-food sources of vitamin C, including citrus fruit and juice, strawberries, tomatoes, red bell peppers, potatoes, and broccoli.

Vitamin D: ✦ Most people get their vitamin D requirement from exposure to sunlight. By spending a short time outside two or three times a week, their bodies are generally able to synthesize all the vitamin D they need. Older people may lose some of the ability to synthesize vitamin D from exposure to sun, and people who live in cold, dark environments may not get enough sunshine. Vitamin D is found naturally in very few foods. But milk, some cereals, and certain breads may be fortified with vitamin D. Foods that naturally contain vitamin D include some fatty fish (herring, salmon, sardines), fish liver oil, and eggs from hens that have been fed vitamin D.

Vitamin E: ✦ Major sources of this vitamin include olive, safflower, and sunflower oils; nuts; whole grains; and leafy green veggies.

Vitamin K: ✦ The dietary form of vitamin K, called phylloquinone, can be found in leafy green vegetables and soybean, cottonseed, canola, and olive oils.

Calcium: ✦ Dairy foods—milk and cheese—provide about 75 percent of the calcium in our diets. Other sources of calcium include yogurt, canned sardines and salmon, pinto and red beans, and tofu. Unfortunately, average dietary intakes of calcium in this country are well below recommended levels for every age and gender group, especially females. For example, only about 10 percent of girls ages 9 to 17 meet calcium recommendations. During the most critical period for developing bone mass, many adolescents are substituting soda for milk. This could have devastating consequences for their later years.

Minerals

Chromium: ✦ Good sources are meat, whole grains, nuts, cheese, and eggs.

Copper: ✦ This mineral is most plentiful in organ meats, shellfish, nuts, and seeds. Wheat bran cereals and whole-grain products are also good sources of copper.

Fluoride: ✦ In the United States, most dietary fluoride is found in drinking water. The fluoride content of most foods is pretty low, less than .05 milligrams per 100 grams, but rich food sources of fluoride include tea, which concentrates fluoride in its leaves, and fish that are eaten with their bones, such as sardines.

Iodine: ✦ The iodine content in most foods depends on the iodine content of the soil in which the food was grown. In addition, seafood is rich in iodine because marine animals can concentrate the iodine from seawater. Certain types of seaweed, for example wakame, are also rich in iodine. Other sources of iodine include iodized salt, cow's milk, navy beans, baked potatoes, and turkey.

Iron: ✦ The amount of iron that is absorbed and used by the body is partly influenced by the iron needs of the individual. Anemic or iron-deficient people absorb a larger proportion of the iron they consume than people who already have sufficient iron stores. The source of the iron also affects how well it can be absorbed by the body. The more readily absorbed form is known as heme iron, which comes from hemoglobin in meat, poultry, and fish. Non-heme iron can be found in eggs and plant foods, such as soy nuts, whole-wheat breads and cereals, bran, apricots, kidney and lima beans, lentils, raisins, prunes and prune juice, tofu, and blackstrap molasses.

National surveys in the United States indicate that the average woman's dietary intake of iron is 12 milligrams per day, and about 15 milligrams per day for pregnant women. But the RDA for women 19–50 is 18 milligrams, 8 milligrams for women 51 and older, 27 milligrams for pregnant women, and 9 milligrams for breast-feeding women. Interestingly enough, men, who don't lose iron each month through menstruation and therefore need less, actually tend to get more than the RDA for iron.

Magnesium: ✦ Because magnesium is part of chlorophyll, which is the green pigment in plants, green leafy vegetables are particularly rich in magnesium. Whole grains and nuts also have a high magnesium content.

Manganese: ✦ This mineral can be found in pineapples, almonds, instant oatmeal, brown rice, lima beans, cooked spinach, sweet potatoes, and green and black tea.

Molybdenum: ✦ Legumes, such as beans, lentils, and peas, are the richest sources of molybdenum, but grain products and nuts are also considered good sources.

Phosphorus: ✦ This mineral is found in most foods because it is a critical component of all living organisms. Dairy products, meat, and fish are particularly rich sources. Phosphorus is also a component of many polyphosphate food additives, and it is present in many soft drinks (particularly colas) as phosphoric acid.

Potassium: ✦ The richest sources of this mineral are fruits and vegetables. Some of the foods with the highest potassium content include bananas, orange juice, artichokes, lima beans, acorn squash, cooked spinach, and sunflower seeds.

Selenium: ✦ The richest food sources of selenium are seafood, liver, kidney, and other organ meats. Grain products also contain modest amounts of selenium, but the soil the grains are grown in determines the actual concentration of the mineral in the food.

Sodium: ✦ Although sodium is necessary for a number of bodily functions, almost no one in this country is sodium-deficient, and most people consume too much, mainly from salt added during food processing or manufacturing. High-salt processed foods include but are certainly not limited to hot dogs, most deli meats, bacon, sausage, dill pickles, tomato juice, ham, canned soups, macaroni and cheese, corned beef hash, chips, cheese curls, crackers, and pretzels, and seasonings such as soy sauce, barbecue sauce, MSG, and ketchup. Remember, a low-salt diet can help prevent hypertension. So look carefully at the sodium content on food labels, and add salt sparingly to meals that you prepare.

Zinc: ✦ Shellfish, beef, and other red meats are rich sources of zinc. Nuts and legumes are relatively good plant sources of this mineral. The fraction of zinc retained and used by the body is relatively high in meat and seafood because of the presence of cysteine and methionine, amino acids that improve zinc absorption.

RDAs, AIs, and NDs: An Explanation

To give you some guidance about what amounts of vitamins and minerals you need to be getting every day, and to enable you to compare those daily requirements with the nutrients listed on the labels of various multivitamin supplements, I've provided a table. The Recommended Dietary Allowances (RDAs, as they are called) provided in Table 8-1 are based on those set by the Food and Nutrition Board of the National Academy of Sciences. In places where I've substituted an AI for an RDA, that indicates that the amount given is an Adequate Intake (AI), a slightly less strong recommendation from the Food and Nutrition Board. For many of the nutrients, I've provided information specific to women in different age groups, and to pregnant and breast-feeding women, too, since their nutrient needs may differ substantially because of the new life they are supporting. The column on the right-hand side of the table provides safe upper limits, which means the maximum daily level that can be consumed without posing any health risk. For some of the nutrients, however, there will be the notation ND, which means that there is no determined recommendation concerning the amount that should be taken or the maximum amount that can be taken safely, because there is insufficient data available so far.

Although many doctors and herbalists may suggest amounts different from those that appear in this table, either for general purposes or to deal with specific health issues, I have chosen to use these recommendations because they represent what I believe to be the best scientific information available to date.

Keep in mind, however, that none of these numbers is set in stone. The science of nutrition is constantly evolving. One example of its evolution is that even as I write this a complete set of new guidelines, called DRIs (Dietary Reference Intakes) is being developed, in response to new information we have gained about the role of nutrients in your health. For now, however, the RDAs are still a valid standard.

Table 8-1 Nutrient Supplements:
What They Do for You and How Much You Need

Nutrient Supplement / Benefits	RDA	Safe Upper Limits (UL)
Vitamin A *An antioxidant essential for vision, growth, reproduction, and immune function. Protects skin and tissues in the mouth, stomach, intestines, and respiratory and urinary tracts from infection. May also help to control blood sugar levels among diabetics.*	*700 mcg; 770 mcg, pregnant women; 1,300 mcg, breast-feeding women*	*1,700 mcg; 3,000 mcg pregnant and breast-feeding women*
Vitamin B$_9$ (folic acid, folate) *Reduces neural tube birth defects by 50 to 80 percent; helps to reduce high blood levels of homocysteine.*	*400 mcg; 600 mcg, pregnant women; 500 mcg, breast-feeding women*	*1,000 mcg*
Vitamin B$_3$ (niacin) *Helps the body to use sugars and fatty acids; helps to produce energy.*	*14 mcg; 18 mcg, pregnant women; 17 mcg, breast-feeding women*	*35 mcg*
Vitamin B$_5$ (pantothenic acid) *Helps body cells to produce energy; small studies suggest it may lower triglycerides and cholesterol.*	*AI: 5 mg; 6 mg, pregnant women; 7 mg, breast-feeding women*	*ND*

Nutrient Supplement / Benefits	RDA	Safe Upper Limits (UL)
Vitamin B$_2$ (riboflavin) *Helps the body to break down sugar and fat for energy; helps to convert niacin to active form.*	1.1 mg; 1.4 mg, pregnant women; 1.6 mg, breast-feeding women	ND
Vitamin B$_1$ (thiamin) *Helps the body to produce energy from carbohydrates.*	1.1 mg; 1.4 mg, pregnant and breast-feeding women	ND
Vitamin B$_6$ (pyridoxine) *Helps the body to fight infection by assisting in the production of antibodies and hemoglobin; helps to produce insulin. May lower risk for cardiovascular diseases, such as heart disease and stroke; research shows it protects against heart disease by lowering homocysteine levels. Other studies show promising evidence for controlling morning sickness.*	1.3 mg; 1.9 mg, pregnant women; 2.0 mg, breast-feeding women	100 mg

Nutrient Supplement / Benefits	RDA	Safe Upper Limits (UL)
Vitamin B$_{12}$ (cobalamin) *Breaks down fat and protein; prevents megaloblastic anemia; may lower risk for cardiovascular diseases, such as heart disease and stroke. May need to be obtained via supplement as you age, because the body loses the ability to absorb it from food. Vegans must also get their B$_{12}$ from a supplement.*	2.4 mg; 2.6 mg, pregnant women; 2.8 mg, breast-feeding women	ND
Biotin *Aids the body in releasing energy from food.*	30 mcg	ND
Vitamin C *An antioxidant that attacks free radicals in the body; shows promise for reducing the risk of heart disease and stroke; may help control blood pressure, prevent chest pain, and keep blood vessels from dilating. It may also keep blood sugar stable in diabetics.*	75 mg; 85 mg, pregnant women; 120 mg, breast-feeding women	2,000 mg

Nutrient Supplement / Benefits	RDA	Safe Upper Limits (UL)
Calcium *Needed for strong bones and teeth. Evidence shows that calcium helps to slow bone loss and osteoporosis associated with aging. Calcium may also reduce systolic blood pressure (upper number) and may reduce your risk of colon cancer. Some studies suggest that taking 1,200 mg/day cuts PMS symptoms in half.*	*AI: 1,000 mg; 1,200 mg, women over 50*	2,500 mg
Chromium *Helps to maintain normal blood sugar and may therefore provide some protection against type II diabetes.*	*25 mcg, women 19–50; 20 mcg, women over 50; 30 mcg, pregnant women; 45 mcg, breast-feeding women*	ND
Copper *Protects against heart abnormalities and cardio-myopathy; needed for healthy connective tissue in the heart and blood vessels. May also help to maintain immune system function.*	*900 mcg; 1,000 mcg, pregnant women; 1,300 mcg, breast-feeding women*	10,000 mcg

Nutrient Supplement / Benefits	RDA	Safe Upper Limits (UL)
Vitamin D *Helps your body to absorb calcium and phosphorus from food; maintains healthy teeth and bones. Reduces risk of osteoporosis, but taken in high doses (above the safe upper limits), it may cause the bone to break down.*	*AI: 5 mcg, women 19–50; 10 mcg, women 50–70; 15 mcg, women over 70*	*50 mcg*
Vitamin E *An antioxidant that may decrease risk of heart attack or death from heart disease by neutralizing free radicals.*	*15 mg; 19 mg, breast-feeding women*	*1,000 mg; 800 mg, breast-feeding women*
Fluoride *Protects against tooth decay by hardening tooth enamel; may also protect against osteoporosis by stimulating new bone formation.*	*AI: 3 mg*	*10 mg*
Iodine *Needed for normal thyroid function.*	*150 mcg; 220 mcg, pregnant women, 290 mcg, breast-feeding women*	*1,100 mcg*

Nutrient Supplement / Benefits	RDA	Safe Upper Limits (UL)
Iron *Protects against anemia; should not be taken in doses higher than the UL, because high doses may contribute to heart disease.*	*18 mg, women 19–50; 8 mg, women over 50; 27 mg, pregnant women; 9 mg, breast-feeding women*	*45 mg*
Vitamin K *Needed for blood clotting and to maintain bone health and kidney function. Should not be taken except under a doctor's care if you're also taking blood thinners.*	*80 mcg*	*30,000 mcg*
Magnesium *Needed for strong bones and teeth, healthy muscles and nerves. May provide some protection against high blood pressure, preeclampsia, heart attack, osteoporosis, migraine headaches, and asthma. Preliminary research suggests a protective effect for PMS symptoms.*	*310 mg, women 19–30; 320 mg, women over 30; 350 mg, pregnant women 19–30; 360 mg, pregnant women over 30; 310 mg, breast-feeding women 19–30; 320 mg, breast-feeding women over 30*	*350 mg*

Nutrient Supplement / Benefits	RDA	Safe Upper Limits (UL)
Manganese *Helps to form bone; involved in helping your body to metabolize cholesterol, carbohydrates.*	AI: 1.8 mg; 2.0 mg, pregnant women, 2.6 mg, breast-feeding women	11 mg
Molybdenum *Helps the body to make hemoglobin. Too much may interfere with the body's ability to absorb copper.*	45 mcg; 50 mcg, pregnant & breast-feeding women	2,000 mcg
Phosphorus *Major component of bones and teeth. Deficiencies are rare, but too much may lower calcium levels in the blood and cause increased bone loss if calcium intake from food is too low to compensate. May prevent muscle weakness and bone pain.*	100 mg	4,000 mg; 3,500 mg, pregnant women

Nutrient Supplement / Benefits	RDA	Safe Upper Limits (UL)
Potassium *Helps body to maintain normal blood pressure. Provides protection against stroke, high blood pressure, osteoporosis, kidney stones. Should be taken only under doctor's care, as taking more than recommended amounts can cause heart problems, particularly in people with kidney disease.*	*ND*	*ND*
Selenium *Helps to maintain immune system function; protects cells from free radicals that can cause heart disease and cancer.*	*55 mcg; 60 mcg, pregnant women; 70 mcg, breast-feeding women*	*400 mcg*
Sodium *Excessive amounts may raise blood pressure and increase the risk for heart disease, hypertension, and stroke. Since there is more in the food supply than is required by the body, there is no minimum level set for sodium.*	*ND*	*ND*

Nutrient Supplement / Benefits	RDA	Safe Upper Limits (UL)
Zinc *Prevents growth retardation in children; maintains immune system integrity; prevents pregnancy complications—low birth weight, premature delivery—in pregnant women; reduces duration of common cold; provides protection against age-related macular degeneration.*	*18 mg; 11 mg, pregnant women; 12 mg, breast-feeding women*	*40 mg*

Who Needs Vitamin and Mineral Supplements?

Probably you, in a word. Why? Because too few people eat the kind of plant-based diet that's needed to reap the kind of optimal health benefits we'd all like. What with busy schedules, kids to raise, elderly parents to care for, careers to manage, and plain survival, good nutrition is one of the first things neglected as we muddle through the maze we call our lives. According to the latest USDA survey, more than 80 percent of women consumed less than two-thirds of the RDA for one or more nutrients.

Our Elders

As we age, our nutritional needs change, because absorption and utilization of certain nutrients become more difficult as the years go by. Older people may therefore have to supplement vitamins C, D, B_6, B_{12}, and folic acid. There may even be a need to supplement zinc and other minerals. Supplementation may also be necessary because some people age 60 and over may lack the financial resources to eat properly. Living on fixed incomes, they sometimes face the difficult choice between food and medicine, or between food and the need to take care of some other pressing obligation. Think about Sister Jones in your church or the senior citizens that you know about in nursing homes (it might even be your own grandmother).

Sistas Starting a Family

If you are even thinking about becoming pregnant, listen up. Folic acid has been proven to prevent serious birth defects in unborn babies. You need 400 mcg of this B vitamin a day to protect your expected bundle of joy, and you need it from the earliest days of pregnancy on, so don't wait until you *know* you're pregnant to be sure you're getting enough of it. An added benefit of folic acid is that it may protect you against heart disease.

Cycling Sistas

Women in general often don't get enough iron, especially during the years before menopause, when we lose so much iron in our menstrual blood, and sistas are no exception. If you still have a menstrual cycle,

What the Science Says

According to the Nurses' Health Study, which examined the dietary intakes of 80,000 nurses, taking a multivitamin for 15 years or more may reduce your risk of colon cancer by 75 percent. Daily doses of multivitamins have been found to cut fetal deaths, low birth weight, and premature births by 40 percent. According to a groundswell of evidence, women with the optimal intake of folate and vitamin B6 may cut their heart disease risk in half compared to women with the lowest intakes of folate. If that's not enough, think about this. Daily multivitamin supplements have been found to boost immune system function by up to 60 percent in elderly people, one of the most vulnerable segments of the population when it comes to disease and infection. One clinical trial suggests that nutritional supplements could cut the rate of infectious disease in half among elderly people. And that's not all. Another study found that elderly people who used vitamins E and C had a 42 percent decreased risk of mortality compared to those who didn't take the vitamins. And there are many other studies suggesting that increased intake of vitamins A, C, E, and other nutrients (some in excess of the RDA) reduces cancer risk, which causes a half million American deaths a year.

Good results are reported almost daily about the

continued

power that can be found in a pill, whether it's calcium's ability to slow down the loss of bone mass in aging adults, vitamin B2's ability to help migraine sufferers and also perhaps prevent cataracts, or the multiple promising effects of niacin, which I'll describe below.

you would do well not only to eat a balanced diet but to take a daily multivitamin/mineral with iron and calcium. See the chart for recommendations about upper levels, however, because amounts too high may contribute to heart disease.

Vegans

If you are the type of vegetarian who eats no eggs or dairy, only fruits, vegetables, nuts, seeds, and grains, you need to supplement your diet with vitamin B_{12}, zinc, and calcium, all nutrients found in great supply in animal foods. You can probably pick up most of your dietary slack by taking a multivitamin daily. There is evidence that multivitamins and vitamin and mineral supplements overall can reduce the risk of disease and expand your life span.

Super Nutrition Supplements with Promise

To say that you can cure all that ails you with nutritional supplements would be a vast oversimplification and, frankly, would be untrue. Still, the science of nutrition is constantly evolving, and every day we learn more about its potential for improving our quality of life. Among all the nutritional supplements that are currently being touted, I've chosen to write about five that I believe show exceptionally strong promise. The evidence for niacin, selenium, and alpha-lipoic acid (ALA) seems compelling. I am also optimistic about the promise of the bioflavonoid quercetin and about a more obscure antioxidant, Pycnogenol. Read on to get a capsule overview of the potential health-promoting benefits of each of these nutrients.

Niacin

Researchers have been investigating the use of niacin to treat a number of different ailments, including migraine headaches, arthritis, diabetes, and high cholesterol. A recent study of arthritis patients found that patients who took daily megadoses of nicotinamide (a form of niacin) for 12 weeks experienced a lessening of symptoms and a 13 percent reduction in the need for medication. In mild to moderate cases of high cholesterol, niacin has been known to rival prescription medications in its effectiveness. Practitioners of both conventional and herbal medicine have had success treating patients with high cholesterol with 2,000-mg doses of niacin (in the form of nicotinic acid). Similarly high doses of niacin, given at the first signs of type I (insulin-dependent) diabetes, appear to help regulate blood sugar and prevent complications of the disease. But no one should consider taking such high doses except under the supervision of a doctor.

Other conditions for which niacin shows promise are circulatory disorders such as Raynaud's disease, intermittent claudication, and maybe tinnitus, a persistent ringing, humming, and buzzing in the ears, that has been linked to poor blood circulation, because the supplement improves circulation by relaxing arteries and veins. Depression, anxiety, and panic disorder may also respond to niacin, because it promotes nerve cell function.

Alpha-Lipoic Acid

Often called the "universal antioxidant," alpha-lipoic acid (ALA) can boost the powers of vitamins C and E and repair cell damage caused by the aging process, which is why dermatologists and cosmeticians often use it topically to improve the appearance of the skin. Studies also show that it can increase insulin levels in diabetics, protect against heart disease and stroke damage, and protect against cancer and maybe memory loss. Some doctors recommend 20–50 milligrams to get protection. Higher doses (up to 300 milligrams) may be needed to control elevated blood sugar in diabetics. A note of caution: At such a high dose, a possible side effect could be headaches.

Selenium

Selenium is a trace mineral that has antioxidant properties. It may protect against cancer and infertility and could give the immune system a boost. Remember, the Daily Value (DV) is 70 micrograms, and the safe Upper Limit (UL) is 200 micrograms. One study found people who took 200 micrograms cut their prostate, lung, and colorectal cancer risk in half. However, as is the case with other nutrients, taking more does not equal greater protection against disease. Taking 1,000 mcg of selenium could prove to be toxic. And mega-doses of 5,000 mcg a day could cause hair loss, diarrhea, abdominal pain, and irritability, so more is not necessarily better and may in fact be much worse.

Pycnogenol

Pycnogenol, the brand name for an extract from pine bark, contains substances that belong to the class of nutrients known as bioflavonoids, which are powerful antioxidants. It may be especially helpful to people with diabetes and hypertension. Because Pycnogenol has anti-inflammatory properties, it reduces blood clotting. Some studies suggest it may potentially stimulate the immune system and be useful in protecting the skin from sun damage. At a dose of 50–100 mg a day, you should reap the potential health-promoting benefits of Pycnogenol without any negative side effects.

Quercetin

This bioflavanoid may reduce allergic reactions to pollen, ragweed, dust, mold, pets, and pollution. Two large studies suggest that quercetin may also reduce coronary heart disease mortality rates and prevent diabetes. Keep a watchful eye for more news about this flavonoid as more research becomes available. To get the protective effect of quercetin, you can take 400–500 milligrams twice a day.

On Taking Precautions: Vitamins and Minerals

Sistas, if you use your supplements wisely, you should be fine. Just remember, there are supplement rules of thumb to keep in mind when you add pills and powders to your diet.

❖ Avoid supplements that provide megadoses. Most cases of nutrient toxicity stem from the use of high-dose supplements. In general, choose a multivitamin/mineral supplement that provides about 100 percent of the Daily Value (DV) of all the vitamins and minerals instead of one that supplies 500 percent DV of one vitamin and only 10 or 20 percent of the DV of another. The exception to this is calcium. You may notice that supplements that contain calcium don't provide 100 percent DV. If they did, the tablets would be too large to swallow.

❖ Check the label for the term *USP*. This ensures that the supplement meets the standards for strength, purity, disintegration, and dissolution established by the testing organization U.S. Pharmacopeia (USP).

❖ Beware of gimmicks. Synthetic vitamins are the same as so-called natural vitamins. Don't be suckered by the promise of added herbs, enzymes, or amino acids—they do nothing but put a hole in your wallet.

❖ Look for expiration dates. Supplements can lose potency over time, especially if you live in a hot and humid climate. If a supplement doesn't have an expiration date, don't buy it. Also, store supplements in a dry, cool place, not the bathroom.

❖ Store your supplements out of the sight and reach of children. Put them in a locked cabinet or other secured location. Don't leave them sitting out on the counter or rely on child-resistant packaging. Be especially careful with any supplements containing iron. Iron overdose is a leading cause of poisoning deaths among children.

❖ Explore your options. If you have difficulty swallowing pills or tablets, ask your doctor whether a chewable or liquid form of the vitamin and mineral supplements might be right for you.

❖ Be safe. Before taking anything other than a standard multivitamin/mineral supplement, check with your doctor, pharmacist, or nutritionist. This is especially important if you have a health problem or are taking prescription medication. High doses of niacin, for instance, can result in liver problems. In addition, supplements may interfere with your medications. Vitamins E and K, for example, aren't recommended if you're taking blood-thinning medications (anticoagulants), because they can complicate the proper control of blood thinning. If you're already taking an individual vitamin or mineral supplement and haven't told your doctor, do so at your next checkup.

Herbs That Can Heal

Some herbal preparations, when used properly and for the right purpose, are particularly beneficial to women. There are also some that women should absolutely avoid.

Women have historically sought herbal concoctions for relief of hormonal changes, whether premenstrually, during menstruation, or after menopause. And for generations it was women who used plants, seeds, roots, barks, and berries to soothe their families' ailments. My grandma Mary was no different. A small-town girl from Orange, Virginia, who married very young and had a big family, she always knew how to make you feel better. If you had a headache, she would tell you to go pick the large "collard-green-looking leaves" that grew in the backyard near her vegetable garden. She would put the leaves in a clean cloth and wrap your head tightly. After a few moments the headache would be lost to those leaves. What the leaves were I don't know, but whenever I have a headache I wish I had asked. Got an upset stomach? No worries—Grandma would come to the rescue after having carefully and lovingly plucked some peppermint from that same garden. She couldn't give you a scientific explanation for why these remedies worked, but she knew they did.

Today, science can explain a lot of what my grandma and maybe yours knew back then. Having hot flashes? Black cohosh may be for you. What about PMS? Try chaste berry, an herb that limits the production of prolactin, a hormone that is a factor in PMS symptoms.

Sounds like a lot of new information, doesn't it? It is, which is why I've prepared a chart describing some of the most commonly used herbs and what they can do for you.

Table 8-2 Herbs and Their Benefits

Herb or Supplement	Benefits
Black cohosh	*Reduces hot flashes in menopausal women; 40 mg is all that is needed. The German Commission E (a regulating body for herbals) recommends that you limit black cohosh use to 6 months or less.*
Chaste berry	*Also called vitex. Relieves symptoms of PMS by reducing prolactin levels and allowing hormones to return to normal balanced levels. Also good for alleviating menopausal symptoms.*
Cramp bark	*Reduces menstrual cramps and provides relief of PMS symptoms.*
Echinacea	*An immune stimulant and an anti-infective. A number of studies have shown it can reduce the length of flulike illnesses if taken at the first sign of illness; two 500 mg tablets can be taken in a dose for up to one week to ward off flulike symptoms. See p. 214 for possible drug interactions.*

Herb or Supplement	Benefits
Feverfew	*Helps reduce migraine headaches and menstrual irregularities. There may be withdrawal symptoms associated with feverfew. You must consume 250 mcg of the active ingredient, parthenolide, to get real benefits.*
Garlic	*Lowers cholesterol and may help to prevent blood clots; preliminary research shows promise for possible cancer prevention; if taken in fresh form, 1 clove taken once a day may result in lowered cholesterol. Remember, do not take garlic in the weeks preceding surgery, as it is a natural blood thinner.*
Ginger	*Used to treat nausea and morning sickness. Powdered capsulated form may be helpful in treating motion sickness.*
Ginkgo biloba	*Increases cerebral blood flow and relieves vertigo. A 1997 study found that ginkgo significantly improved cognitive functioning in some patients with Alzheimer's. Herbalists recommend taking 80 mg of standardized ginkgo biloba extract. See p. 215 for possible drug interactions.*

Herb or Supplement	Benefits
Ginseng root	*Increases the ability to handle both physical and emotional stress. Herbalists recommend taking 1,000 mg three times a day for up to three months. A cautionary note: All ginseng is not created equal. Some brands may contain little of the active ingredient that provides health benefits. Use only standardized preparations from reputable companies. See p. 303 for possible drug interactions.*
Kava kava	*A natural sedative used in the Pacific islands for years to treat anxiety, pain, and muscle tightness. Has diuretic benefits (meaning it releases water from the body). If used over an extended period, it can lead to yellow discoloration of the skin. See p. 303 for possible drug interactions.*
Milk thistle	*May help people with liver problems, including hepatitis B and C and cirrhosis.*
Peppermint oil	*A menthol-rich oil from the leaves of the peppermint plant. Aids in digestion and may relieve irritable bowel syndrome; peppermint tea is good for cramping. Peppermint tea is not good for young children, as the menthol sensation may cause choking.*
Red raspberry	*Uterine tonic; helps to nourish uterine smooth muscle and to reduce menstrual cramps.*

Herb or Supplement	Benefits
Valerian root	*Helpful with PMS. Reduces anxiety and provides a sedative effect to promote sound sleep. Also acts as a muscle relaxant. Herbalists recommend taking 150–300 mg of standardized extract.*

Note: These are suggestions for herbal remedies that may potentially alleviate certain health problems as described in the above chart. However, you should consult an experienced herbalist for treatment before taking any herbal remedy.

Herbs That Can Harm

Some herbs can work for you, but there are many that may work against you, especially if you are a woman, and in some instances especially if you are a pregnant woman.

Aloe
Aloe is usually found in the form of a gel that can be used on the skin, but it can also be found in liquid form. It is a very powerful laxative and should not be taken internally by pregnant women, children, or the elderly.

Chaparral
Sometimes called creosote, this herb comes from an olive-green shrub that grows in the southwestern United States. It is touted as a cancer and anti-aging

remedy, but beware. It causes acute hepatitis, and the FDA has strongly recommended against its use.

Comfrey

This wild flowering plant has been known to cause liver cancer in lab animals. It is generally used externally to help heal broken bones and wounds. It is used internally as a tea to heal stomach ulcers. Since several cases of liver cancer have been reported with comfrey use, the American Herbal Products Association has recommended that it not be used at all.

The Folate Failure

A national campaign kicked off in 1992 by the U.S. Public Health Service recommended that women of childbearing age consume 400 micrograms of folic acid a day to reduce the incidence of spina bifida and other neural tube defects in their babies. Since folic acid is important during the earliest days of pregnancy, this recommendation should be followed by all women in that age range, not just women who know that they are pregnant. A Centers for Disease Control and Prevention survey found that the campaign has been largely successful—except among black women. While there has been a roughly threefold increase in folate consumption among women in other groups, African American women had the lowest folate concentrations of all the study's participants.

Dong Quai

Also known as angelica, dong quai is usually taken for relief from menopausal symptoms, but it should not be used if you experience a heavy menstrual cycle, since it can increase bleeding, and also should not be used if there's any chance you're pregnant. Overdosage can have negative effects on blood pressure, heart rhythm, and respiration.

Pennyroyal

A member of the mint family, pennyroyal is commonly used as a natural abortion aid. It is known to be highly toxic and extremely dangerous. It causes severe hemorrhaging. In one case, a woman who took only 2 tablespoons of the extract hemorrhaged and died within two hours.

Sassafras

The FDA banned the use of sassafras in root beer back in 1970. You've probably heard about older women in our community making sassafras tea for stomach comfort. That's because it's thought to be an anti-spasmodic. But according to the FDA, safrole, a substance in the oil of the sassafras tree, has caused liver damage and lung cancer in rats.

Weight Loss and Fitness Supplements

Cascara Bark

Often used as a laxative, cascara bark is also used by some as a weight loss aid. However, in my opinion, it is best avoided altogether, especially by pregnant and nursing women. Since breast milk retains the active ingredients in cascara bark, the herb can harm babies. Brewed up in a tea as a weight loss aid, and usually mixed with some other diuretic, too, it can cause dramatic fluid loss, which will indeed result in temporary weight loss. But the weight loss comes at a hefty price, because when most people take it for this purpose they drink up to a quart a day of the tea, and in these amounts the resulting loss of water and potassium can cause the heart to stop beating.

Creatine Monohydrate

Viewed as a "legal" steroid, creatine is generally used by athletes to increase endurance and performance during high-intensity exercise. Body builders and fitness competitors often use it. Creatine increases body mass (sometimes by as much as 2 to 6 pounds in as little as one week). But this weight gain is probably due more to the water that is held in muscles than to actual increases in lean muscle mass. Since the jury is still out in terms of long-term study of this supplement, the general public is warned against its use. To date, there is little information available on side effects, although there is concern about creatine supplementation at high doses because it is excreted by the kidneys. Consult a registered dietitian, sports nutritionist, or doctor before trying this or any supplement.

Ephedra

Low doses of ephedra (or ephedrine, its active ingredient) were originally used to treat asthma and allergies, but then it took off as a weight loss aid. If you've ever seen the *Heart & Soul* TV show or read any of my columns or stories in *Heart & Soul* magazine or on BET.com, you know I don't recommend the use of ephedra. This is a big disappointment to many folks who want a quick fix to weight loss. But now that the FDA has reported at least 100 ephedra-related deaths and issued strict warnings against its use for weight loss, I cannot possibly get behind this supplement. Women are at particular risk for stroke when using the amounts of ephedra commonly found in weight loss supplements, and there is evidence that it could be harmful to anyone with high blood pressure or a predisposition to heart disease. Yes, it is an appetite suppressant, which causes you to eat less, and yes, it is a diuretic, which promises water weight loss. But you'd prefer to get the weight off and be alive and in good health, right? So take my advice and steer clear of this one. Clearly, the benefits are not worth the risk.

Pyruvate

Pyruvate, a natural by-product of the body's metabolism, has shown some promise as a weight loss aid, slightly boosting the body's ability to burn fat and calories. One study found that supplementing with 20 grams of pyruvate daily in combination with very-low-calorie diets (1,000 calories) netted very modest results. Study participants saw only small increases in weight loss, 2 to 3 pounds over a three-week period. But the results from another group of researchers were more encouraging. They observed a 2.6-pound weight loss over six weeks in their participants. After participants took 6 grams of pyruvate on a 2,000-calorie diet and exercised regularly, researchers observed small improvements when they compared the weight loss to a control group. Scientists say these weight loss results may be minor but that over time they could prove to be just the ticket for motivating people to stick with their plans and adopt healthier lifestyles. They recommend 3–5 grams of pyruvate daily for gradual weight loss but caution against its use on an empty stomach for ulcer sufferers.

Natural Versus Harmless

As I said before, just because they're derived from natural sources doesn't mean that herbal products can't harm you. Tobacco is a plant, and so is the coca from which cocaine is made, but the last time I checked they were both capable of doing a lot of harm. Don't fall for the "natural" terminology prominently displayed on labels, thinking it means you're in good hands. Educate yourself before taking any herbal supplement, and make sure you check with a bona fide herbalist who knows about the herbal product you're considering. Also make sure you tell your doctor anytime you're taking any supplement because it might have an effect on the nutrients you're getting from food or on medications that you need for other health reasons. Finally, don't abandon prescription medicines in favor of herbal remedies until you've fully researched the subject, checked with your doctor and/or nutritionist, and armed yourself with enough information to make a solid decision.

On Taking Precautions: Herbs

Clearly, there are many herbs and botanicals that are beneficial to women. But be careful: Only use herbal remedies and preparations when you know the credentials of the expert who designed them, and know what and how much you are taking. Talk to your physician to make sure any herbs you take don't interfere with other medications. Also, if you are pregnant, you shouldn't take herbal products. There are too many potentially harmful effects on the baby growing inside you to take the risk.

Recently, the Food and Drug Administration has issued warnings and recalls for several herbal products. But the herbal industry is relatively unregulated. The problem? The Dietary Supplement Health and Education Act, which was passed in 1994, does not include an FDA requirement that manufacturers of herbs prove their products are safe or effective before marketing them. Instead it simply suggests that companies police themselves and disclose information to consumers. This has left the manufacturers of herbal products free to make general health claims on their labels.

Though experts say most herbs are safe when taken as directed, a series of recent reports underscore the danger behind the loose herbal industry regulations. Some herbals can cause relatively minor problems; if you stop taking feverfew, for example, you might experience withdrawal symptoms. Long-term use of kava kava can lead to a yellowish discoloration of your skin. But a small number of herbal products have led to liver damage, seizures, heart attacks, stroke, and even death. As you read earlier, ephedra has resulted in over 100 deaths. And many of the adverse effects caused by herbal products occur in interaction with other medications, allergies, impurities, or when taken in dangerously high doses.

Herbal Remedies on a Collision Course: Herb-Drug Interactions

Because herbal remedies are not regulated by the FDA, unless you are careful to buy standardized extracts it's often hard to tell how much of the herb's active ingredient is contained in a given product. Also, there are a number of circumstances in which you need to be careful about mixing herbs with other medications. So you should always let your doctor know what you're taking if you're being given a prescription medication. And if you're going in for surgery and will be put under sedation or anesthesia, it is vital that you tell the anesthesiologist what you're taking. Take a look at a few of the more common prescription drug–herb mismatches that could do you in.

Echinacea
I know many of you take echinacea to ward off colds and to build your immune system, but because echinacea is an immunostimulant, it may alter the effects of anabolic steroids, amiodarone (Cordarone), alprazolam (Xanax), methotrexate (Rheumatrex), ketoconazole (Nizoral), and cyclosporine (Sandimmune). So be very careful.

Ephedra

This is a dangerous and risky supplement, especially when combined with other medications. When combined with decongestants such as pseudoephedrine (found in Actifed, Dristan, Sinutab, Sudafed, and others) or stimulants such as caffeine, ephedra may cause sedation, heart attack, seizures, and even death.

Ginkgo Biloba

Ginkgo increases to the anticoagulant effect of aspirin, clopidogrel (Plavix), dipyridamole (Persantine), ticlopodine (Ticlid), and warfarin (Coumadin), which may lead to spontaneous and excessive bleeding.

Ginseng

Ginseng can set off a number of interactions. When mixed with warfarin (Coumadin), it can lead to excessive bleeding. With phenelzine (Nardil) it can cause headache, trembling, and manic behavior. Since ginseng may cause rapid heartbeat and hypertension, it should never be mixed with digoxin (Lanoxin), which is a heart medication used to regulate heartbeat.

Kava Kava

Since kava kava is known as a sedative, it should not be taken with other sedatives, sleeping pills, antipsychotics, alcohol, alprazolam (Xanax), drugs that treat Parkinson's disease, or anesthetics. In combination with some of these other medications, it could result in deep sedation or even coma.

St. John's Wort

Much touted as an antidepressant, St. John's wort can interfere with the effectiveness of medications for HIV/AIDS and certain cancers. It can also result in seizures.

Frequently Asked Questions

Q Dr. Ro: When is the best time to take a multivitamin?

A *As long as you take a high-quality multivitamin, it doesn't matter what time of day you take it. You should, however, try to take your supplement with a meal. In the best of all possible worlds, you would take your supplement in several divided doses throughout the day. This helps maximize your body's ability to absorb and use the nutrients in the supplement. But that would require breaking your tablets into pieces and taking a piece with each meal, which can be inconvenient and difficult to remember. It's better to take your multivitamin in its one-dose form than not to take one at all.*

Q Dr. Ro: Some say antioxidants are the closest thing to a cure-all on the market; others say all I need is a balanced diet. I'm confused by all this information.

A *You're not alone in your confusion. I have clients coming to me all the time telling me they're swallowing handfuls of antioxidants such as vitamins A, C, and E and beta-carotene. They're convinced if they just take enough of these in high enough doses, they can ride the quick bus to good health—undo the damage from too many trips to KFC, reverse the aging process, and maybe even live forever! My clients believe this information because they've heard that antioxidants neutralize free radicals, those unstable oxygen molecules that, left unchecked, can damage cells, causing cancer and heart disease. And even though antioxidants can be found in whole foods, such as broccoli and oranges, they choose to go the pill route instead of the food route because it's quicker and, they believe, easier.*

Hogwash. And government scientists convened by the Institute of Medicine agree with me, coming down firmly on the whole-foods side in the food-pill debate. But every day a new study touting the benefits of pills crops up, leaving consumers like you bothered and bewildered.

Here's the science behind the controversy. Some studies say pills have worked wonders against disease. A daily dose of 400 to 800 IU of vitamin E has been shown in one study to reduce heart attack risk by 77 percent in people with atherosclerosis. But another study found that people who took megadoses of vitamin E for five years suffered just as many strokes and heart attacks as those taking placebos. Perhaps those doses were too high, as a number of studies have found that megadoses of antioxidants in pill form can actually do more harm than good.

The long and short of it is, we know that eating more fruits and vegetables, which are loaded with natural antioxidants, will reduce your risk of certain diseases. And when you eat antioxidant-rich foods you get additional

disease fighters—other vitamins, minerals, and fiber—
as part of the package. Dietary supplements are meant
to supplement an already healthful diet, not replace
foods you need to eat every day. Bottom line? For maximum nutritional benefits, scarf down those fruits and
vegetables, and supplement with a multivitamin containing antioxidants and minerals.

Q Dr. Ro: My HMO has started providing cov-
erage for some alternative therapies, including herbal medication. Doesn't this mean
taking herbal supplements is safe?

A Herbal remedies are incredibly popular.
Americans spent $591 million on them in
2000. The number of people using complementary therapies—inlcuding herbal medicine, massage, megadoses
of vitamins and minerals, folk remedies, and homeopa-
thy—jumped from 33 percent in 1990 to more than 42
percent in 1997, according to the NIH's National
Center for Complementary and Alternative Medicine.
Despite this popularity, however, there are limits to what
herbal supplements can do. Get a medical diagnosis of
your ailment and talk to your doctor before taking any
herbal remedies. If you have a serious condition, an
herbal remedy probably isn't the best choice. If you are
pregnant or breast-feeding, don't use herbal supplements. And don't mix herbals and prescription medications without medical supervision.

Q   Dr. Ro: Should I stop taking my herbal supplement before having surgery?

A   *The main cause for concern for surgical patients using herbs is excessive bleeding. According to the American Society of Anesthesiologists, ginkgo biloba and feverfew may reduce the number of platelets in the blood and thus interfere with blood clotting. Other herbs also reported to inhibit clotting include garlic, ginger, ginseng, dong quai, and danshen. In addition, some herbs may intensify or prolong the effects of narcotic drugs and anesthesia. Problematic herbs in this category include valerian, kava kava, and St. John's wort.*

You should stop taking all herbs two to three weeks prior to any surgery. If time does not allow for that, bring whatever you have been taking to the surgeon and anesthesiologist so they can evaluate the risks.

Secret

The Food Guide Pyramid
May Get You Only Halfway There

 And God populated the earth with broccoli and cauliflower and spinach and green and yellow vegetables of all kinds, so Man and Woman would live long and healthy lives. And Satan created fast food. And the fast-food industry brought forth the 99-cent double cheeseburger. And Satan said to Man, "You want fries with that?" And Man said, "Yes, supersize them!" And Man and Woman and all their children grew to massive proportions, and . . . well, you know how this story ends if you don't decide to do something about it.

Solving the Mysteries of the
Food Guide Pyramid

The Food Guide Pyramid has been in existence since 1992, yet as I travel the country speaking to thousands of African American women, look at the hundreds of letters and e-mails I receive, and listen to the voices at the other end of the phone line, the question is always "What should I be eating"? This tells me that the Food Guide Pyramid, as a tool for eating and dietary guidance, has eluded most of the people in my audience. Today, we are still as confused as ever about the all-important questions of what to eat and how much of it we should eat in order to be healthy. So it's not surprising that record numbers of us are overweight and obese.

The Food Guide Pyramid was developed to help Americans simplify their dietary dilemma by telling them what to eat in a format that would, at least theoretically, eliminate the necessity to calculate the number of calories and amount of nutrients in their foods. Once scientists had determined the Recommended Dietary Allowances (RDAs), amounts of vitamins and minerals necessary to prevent deficiency diseases, they had the information they needed to provide the public with a detailed guide to healthy eating in terms of calories and units of nutrients. But since having to think about food choices in such a technical way isn't very practical for ordinary folks, in 1980 the U.S. Department of Agriculture (USDA) and the Department of Health and Human Services (HHS) assembled an expert panel of scientists whose job it was to simplify the task of making nutritionally sound food choices. They eventually developed the Food Guide Pyramid, which was considered a breakthrough development at the time. Until then, the only official advice we'd been given about how to eat was to choose from among the four basic food groups. Never before had consumers received such relatively specific dietary advice. But here we are two decades later, fatter than ever and suffering from a veritable epidemic not just of obesity but of type II diabetes, a mainly preventable disease. What went wrong?

What Has the Pyramid Done for You Lately?

Yes, it's true that we didn't follow the advice we were given. While many Americans may be familiar with the pyramid, it seems they are not willing to use it as the guide it was designed to be. African Americans in particular seem to lack a working knowledge of what it is and how to use it. According to the USDA's Healthy Eating Index (HEI), a measure of people's dietary quality, African Americans get low marks for their dietary habits. As summarized in a USDA study, data from the years 1994–1996 reveal that black folks have a "particularly poor quality" diet. The HEI is broken into 10 components. Components 1–5 measure the degree to which a person's diet conforms to the Food Guide Pyramid's serving suggestions for the five major food groups. In other words, if the Pyramid suggests that we eat 6 to 11 daily servings of grains, the survey looks at whether we do or don't eat that many servings. Other recommendations from the Pyramid regarding food groups and the number of servings within each one are 3 to 5 servings of vegetables; 2 to 4 servings of fruits; 2 to 3 servings of milk, yogurt, and cheese; and 2 to 3 servings of meat and protein. Oils, fats, and sweets should be used sparingly each day. Components 6 through 10 of the Healthy Eating Index measure total fat and saturated fat consumption, cholesterol and sodium intakes, and the variety in a person's diet.

African Americans had an overall score of 59 on a 0–100 scale, compared to a score of 64 for whites and a score of 65 for other racial groups. Only 5 percent of African Americans had a good diet, compared to 11 percent of whites. While the vast majority of people in all groups could use some improvement in their diets, 28 percent of black folks have a "poor diet," compared to 16 percent of whites and 14 percent of other racial groups. The one bright spot in this report is that we are beginning to get it when it comes to consuming too much cholesterol. The degree to which African Americans have their total cholesterol under control is reflected in the score of 7.4 on a scale of 0–10. But on getting enough fruit in our diets, we fail miserably. Our score was the lowest mean score of all our scores for any foods, a pitiful 3.5. It is understandable that our score for milk consumption would be low (the second lowest of all our scores), in that 75 percent of black people reportedly have lactose intolerance. But we also score worse than other groups on total fat and saturated fat consumption. A mere 31 percent of African Americans meet the dietary recommendation for keeping total fat at or below the recommended level. In fact, fewer than half of black people meet the dietary recommendations for 9 out of 10 of the HEI categories. What does that say to you? Clearly, we ain't using the Pyramid to guide our food choices.

Even if we did, I am not sure it is to our benefit to do so. Some experts agree that while the Food Guide Pyramid might have been a good attempt at getting

America to eat better, it's inadequate as a prescription for good health. Why?

The Base of the Pyramid Stands on Shaky Ground

Think about it this way. The Pyramid is supposed to be built like the pyramids in Egypt. Symbols of power, they rest on a base that provides them with stability and strength. Only this pyramid may have a questionable foundation. At its base, you are encouraged to eat more foods from the grains group—that's breads, cereals, pasta, and rice. However, the Food Guide Pyramid doesn't specify what *kind* of grains we should be eating, mainly whole grains. Nor does it make it clear that the 6 to 11 servings that are recommended represent a range or that *where* on that range you would locate the appropriate number of servings for yourself depends on your height, weight, and activity level. For example, an overweight, sedentary woman who's five feet two inches tall should *not* be eating 11 servings of grains, even of healthy whole grains, while a lean, active man who's six-two might do just fine consuming that amount of carbohydrates.

To date, it seems that most people have interpreted the Pyramid's grain recommendation to mean that it's okay to eat 6 to 11 servings a day of white bread, white rice, pasta, and sugar-laden refined-grain cereals. That's probably not what scientists intended when they made this recommendation initially. In the 1980s, when many nutritionists and doctors thought of meat and fat as the enemy, encouraging people to eat more breads and cereals probably seemed like a great idea. Even today, it might be fairly good advice if it just specified that you need to make sure that most of those grains are whole! Eating fewer white-bread-type foods is of particular importance to us because, as I explained in Secret 2, African Americans may be predisposed to obesity on account of the thrifty gene. Since the refined carbohydrates encouraged at the base of the Pyramid are low-fiber foods and are generally served with high-fat sauces, butter, and toppings, they easily lead to weight gain.

Further, they are usually eaten in gargantuan portions. C'mon, when was the last time you ate a serving of pasta that didn't really amount to at least two (or three) servings? You know it's true. Let me also remind you that the body processes these refined carbs much quicker than their whole-grain counterparts, which means that insulin levels spike, removing glucose from the blood with such ravenousness that you get hungry again very soon after eating. Simply put, you are more likely to put on excess pounds by eating white bread, pasta, and rice than on the whole-grain versions of those foods. A person whose body may already be genetically programmed by the thrifty gene to hold on to that weight should make a point of cutting back on these refined grains.

The Next Level

Moving up from the base of the Pyramid to the next level, you're encouraged to eat more fruits and vegetables—three to five servings of vegetables, two to four of fruits. What's wrong with this picture?

Current scientific thinking suggests that because of the health benefits of eating more vegetables and fruit, which help to protect you against chronic disease, these foods should at the very least be sharing the base of the Pyramid with whole grains, not appearing on the next level. Whether you are trying to achieve weight loss or weight maintenance, you stand a better chance of realizing your goal by eating *more* fruits and vegetables and *fewer* of the bread, cereal, and pasta products that currently occupy the base of the Pyramid. In a nutshell, my biggest problem with the Pyramid is that at a time when we're a fatter nation than ever before, and black folks are suffering and dying needlessly from preventable diseases, this plan may well add to our plight.

Further, if three-quarters of African Americans are lactose-intolerant, the recommended two to three servings of milk, yogurt, and cheese should at least include an advisory about substituting lactose-modified foods or taking one of the lactose-digesting aids (which you can now buy at drugstores and grocery stores) before eating from the dairy group. A recommendation about eating low-fat versions of these foods would also be a good idea. And for those people who just don't want to eat dairy, it should be noted that you can get calcium from calcium-fortified orange juice or soy milk, tofu processed with calcium sulfate (a half cup contains almost as much calcium as a cup of skim milk), and canned fish eaten with its bones, such as salmon and sardines. Although some leafy greens such as spinach and collards contain calcium, be forewarned that they are not a good source of calcium because they also contain substances called oxalates, which bind themselves to minerals such as calcium and interfere with the body's ability to absorb and use the minerals.

Another place I find fault with the Food Guide Pyramid is in the level where it recommends two to three servings of meat, poultry, fish, and eggs. I'd recommend including soy products—soy milk, soybeans, soy nuts, tofu, textured vegetable protein—as a frequent alternative source of protein. But soy doesn't even get mentioned in the USDA Pyramid.

Finally, if we are truly to get serious about our eating habits, we must consider once and for all how to prepare the foods we recommend that people consume. That said, the Food Guide Pyramid has nothing to say about fresh herbs or spices we can use to season our foods. We're simply told to use the fats, oils, and sugars at the top of the Pyramid "only in moderation"—but we're given no advice about how to make our food taste good in the absence of those substances.

According to what you tell me, not only do you want to know which foods to eat and how much of them to eat, but you need to know what to put on those foods so that you can eat them with pleasure but without gaining weight. For this reason, to my mind any dietary system should make recommendations to enhance food flavors. In addition to herbs and spices, there are juices from vegetables and fruits that add tremendous flavor and also have nutritional value on their own merits.

Blackening Up the Pyramid

Yes, I've seen the Soul Food Pyramid, and no, I don't think it's much different from the traditional mainstream version. Although I'm certainly a fan of specific soul foods cooked in healthful ways, as I discussed in Secret 4, the only difference I've been able to detect between the standard Food Guide Pyramid and the Soul Food Pyramid is that the latter may contain collard greens in the vegetables section—no doubt cooked with plenty of bacon grease or ham hock fat—and corn bread in the grains category. Still, the basic structure is the same. So what, then, is the answer?

Dr. Ro's Color Plate System

There is growing evidence that eating a more colorful plant-based diet sustains life and longevity better than the traditional model we have of the brown and beige meat-and-potatoes diet that got us to where we are today—Fat City. My color plate system is a very basic, no-nonsense system of eating that requires no calculation and no counting of calories or fat grams, and removes the guesswork from your meal plan. It focuses on the consumption of ample quantities of fresh fruits and vegetables, soy, and whole grains—many of which are traditional staples with origins in our African homeland. My meal plan is based on three meals and three snacks a day with endless and delicious food choices.

First, let's talk about the colors. There are five color families from which you'll be choosing your fruits and vegetables: red, purple, green, orange, and yellow. Here is a list of the color families and some of the foods within each:

Red: tomatoes, red bell peppers, beets, radishes, apples, strawberries, watermelon, cherries, red grapefruit, pomegranates

Purple: blackberries, blueberries, eggplant, radicchio, raisins, grapes

Green: collard greens, kale, broccoli, mustard greens, spinach, edamame (green soybeans), creesy salad, cabbage, turnip greens, brussels sprouts, green beans, green peas

Orange: pumpkin, mango, orange bell peppers, sweet potato, carrots, oranges, apricots, nectarines, papaya, peaches, butternut squash

Yellow: summer squash, yellow bell peppers, pineapple, lemon, guava, bananas.

Nutrient Contribution of Color Groups

Each color plate category contains foods of a certain color and the nutrients tend to be found in each of the color groups. For example, the *red plate group* contains foods that are rich in antioxidants such as lycopene and vitamins A and C. The *purple plate group* includes foods rich in antioxidants such as anthocyanins, which protect against heart disease. Many of the foods in the *green plate group* are rich in carotenoids such as lutein and zeaxanthin (which are good for your eyes) and other chemical compounds such as isothiocyanate and indoles (which protect against cancer). The *orange plate group* contains foods that have high levels of cancer-preventing carotenoids. Many of them are also rich in vitamin A, which contributes to eye health. The *yellow plate group* contains foods rich in potassium, antioxidants such as vitamin A, and carotenoids, good for your eye health. And besides the various phytonutrients specific to individual groups, the fiber contributed by most of these fruits and vegetables helps in the protection against diabetes, heart disease and other circulatory diseases, and all kinds of bowel problems ranging from constipation to irritable bowel syndrome.

At the end of the day, you want to have created designer meals, where by design—nature's and yours—you have a plate that includes as many of these colors as possible, all adding up to meals that are as tasty as they are nutritious, and beautiful to boot. All fruits and vegetables in all colors belong on your plate. The nutrients I've listed as being specific to each color group represent just the beginnings of what we will be learning about phytochemicals and their benefits in years to come.

Combining Colors to Make the Perfect Meal

I've presented my eating plan on plates because we don't eat on Pyramids, but we do eat our food on plates. By showing you what a nutritionally well-designed plate of food looks like, my color plate system is meant to help you derive maximum nutritional benefit from the foods you eat, with minimal effort and planning. All you have to think about is creating meals that include foods from as many of the various color groups as possible. So an ideal day would consist of meals that include foods that are green, yellow, red, purple, and orange. When you have done this and added whole grains, low-fat protein sources like beans and soy, small amounts of lean meats, fish, chicken, turkey, and nuts, and the healthful and delicious seasonings that I recommend, you have got the Dr. Ro Color Plate System down. I'll say more about the proportions in which the foods are to be eaten, and portion sizes, below.

Soy: Soybeans and Tofu

My color plate system does include small amounts of lean chicken, turkey, meat, and fish for protein. But I want you to consider trying another low-fat form of protein food that goes a step further toward protecting you from chronic disease. That's soy. Not just for the woman trying to dodge hot flashes and night sweats, no ma'am. Soy is for just about anyone who wants to cut calories and ward off disease. The isoflavones in soy, such as genistein and daidzein, are antioxidants that combat cellular damage and may help the immune system fight off cancer cells. Soy also provides a high-quality source of protein, fiber, iron, and bone-strengthening calcium.

Soybeans: ✦ Since I know many of you may resist eating tofu or drinking soy milk, let's look at the nutritional benefits of soybeans, which you can find in the frozen food department and many produce sections of most grocery stores these days and which are as compulsively snackable as any of those salty junk foods on the market—and much lower in calories.

The fiber first: In these tiny nutritional powerhouses,

you can find soluble fiber, which protects against heart disease, and insoluble fiber, which speeds up the intestinal tract, aiding in elimination and keeping carcinogenic (cancer-causing) agents from making a home in your intestines and increasing your risk of cancer. Soybeans also contain a good amount of calcium and iron, two minerals especially found in short supply in black women's diets, and of B vitamins, magnesium, and zinc.

Table 9-1 Calcium and Isoflavone Content of Commonly Consumed Soy Foods

Food	Isoflavones	Calcium
Soy milk, 1 cup	40 mg	80 mg
Fortified soy milk, 1 cup	40 mg	200–300 mg
Tofu, ½ cup	40 mg	130 mg
Prepared TVP, ½ cup	35 mg	85 mg
Soybeans, mature, ½ cup	35 mg	80 mg
Soybeans, green (edamame), ½ cup	35 mg	130 mg
Soy nuts, 1 ounce	40 mg	130 mg

Tofu: ✦ Tofu is made from soy milk in a process that resembles making yogurt or cheese. It's a great source of protein, lower in fat than most animal sources of protein, and of course completely free of saturated fat, the unhealthy kind of fat in animal products. Soy milk has no natural calcium, but many kinds of tofu are good sources of calcium because the process by which most tofu is made uses a calcium compound.

No longer an exotic food, tofu can be found in ordinary grocery stores as well as in health food markets, in the Asian markets where you may be accustomed to buying much of your produce if you live in a big city, or in specialty Chinese and Japanese markets.

The most common kind comes in soft, firm, and extra-firm varieties. I'd recommend starting with firm. This is the standard cooking tofu, good for frying, sautéing, stir-frying, and grilling. In the grocery store it's sold in water-packed, refrigerated cartons. In health food and Asian stores you may find it floating in large tubs of water. If the store does a high volume of business so you know there's a frequent turnover, if you trust the cleanliness of the market, and if the water and the tofu itself smell fresh and sweet, then buying it straight from one of those tubs can offer you a particularly delicious and economical form of tofu. If not, stick with the packaged, refrigerated tofus, many of which are also excellent.

When using water-packed tofu, it's best to let it drain on paper towels for a little while. Otherwise the tofu may release water into the dish you're cooking it in, diluting the flavors. Some cooks even press the tofu for half an hour or so, covering it with aluminum foil or a clean dish cloth and putting a cutting board on top of it, with an iron skillet or a large can to weigh it down.

This is probably necessary only if you're going to deep-fry the tofu, because if you don't the water in it could spatter up from the oil and potentially burn you.

Silken tofu has an almost custardy texture. It's also available in different firmnesses—soft, firm, and extra firm—but it's generally more delicate than the other kind and is particularly useful puréed for sauces, dips, mock cream soups, salad dressings, flavored mayonnaise substitutes, and fruit smoothies. It is sold in aseptically sealed cartons that need no refrigeration until they are opened.

Textured Vegetable Protein (TVP): ✦ TVP is a meaty-tasting soy product made from defatted soy flour. It is a credible low-fat meat substitute that may help you to ease more soy into your diet. Use it in spaghetti "meat" sauce, "meatloaf," or any recipe that uses ground meat. TVP is readily available in most health food stores, in some supermarkets, and by direct mail order through the Archer Daniels Midland Corporation, which holds the TVP trademark. You might try healthyeating.com as an alternative source.

Nuts to You

Another potential source of protein that would be a good replacement for some of the meats you currently eat, which are loaded with saturated fat and cholesterol, is the nut family. Unlike soy, nuts are at least mentioned in the Food Guide Pyramid as one of the possible sources of protein, but nowhere is there any indication that they might be preferable to a steak in their impact on your health. Not only are nuts rich in protein, but they provide a better form of fat—monounsaturated fat instead of the saturated fat in all animal products—which helps protect you from heart disease and other chronic illnesses. Some nuts, such as almonds and walnuts, are particularly rich in the healthy omega-3 fatty acids. Many nuts are also rich sources of fiber, minerals such as potassium and magnesium, and vitamins such as vitamin E.

Just 1 ounce of nuts a day—a scant handful—has protective health effects. Some studies have found that people who eat nuts frequently have lower rates of heart disease than people who rarely eat nuts. Of the 84,000 women in the Harvard Nurses' Health Study, those who ate nuts five times a week had a 35 percent lower risk of heart disease. (I should note that their nut consumption included peanuts, members of the class of plants called legumes, which are not actually nuts.) There is also mounting evidence that adding nuts to your diet can help prevent diabetes. And stay tuned for more research on the health effects of nuts on blood pressure and cancer. Just make sure the nuts you choose are lightly salted or, better yet, salt-free, and be careful to eat them only in modest amounts, because they're relatively high in calories, as you can see below. Still, they make a better choice for a between-meal snack than a candy bar or a bag of chips, and some cuisines make them part of main courses instead of meat or chicken. You might try doing the same, perhaps by adding some walnuts, watercress or spinach, and grated Parmesan cheese to whole-wheat pasta.

Table 9-1 How Many Nuts Make a Serving?

Nut	Serving Size	Calories per Serving
Soy nuts	¼ cup	120
Almonds	22 nuts	170
Brazil nuts	6–8 nuts	185
Cashews	18 nuts	160
Hazelnuts	20 nuts	175
Macadamia nuts	10–12 nuts	200
Peanuts	28 nuts	165
Pecans (halves)	20 nuts	200
Pistachio nuts (shelled)	47 nuts	160
Walnuts (halves)	14 nuts	185

What's on the Plate?

Now let's talk about the serving size of the foods on your plate, and the relative proportions of the various foods. I said earlier that you'd have to change your mind in order to change your waistline. The new mind-set means not only putting less of certain foods on the plate, but reorganizing the plate, too. You've no doubt heard the expression "If you want to lose weight, push back from the plate." Well, if you make the plate changes I'm suggesting, pushing back from it may not even be necessary.

How do you reorganize your plate—and your thinking? By covering the plate with foods in the reverse of the way you eat now. Take dinner, for example. When you sit down to dinner, you are likely to put more meat than vegetables or grains on the plate, right? What probably happens is that your steak, chop, or chicken is close to 8 or 10 ounces, while you might serve up a smidgen of greens and a whole lot of whipped potatoes. Do I know what's happening in your dietary life or what? If you eat at a restaurant, it's even worse. You might have up to 16 ounces of meat on that plate with those whipped potatoes (topped with mounds of butter) and maybe a creamed vegetable. Think about what that must add up to in calories and fat.

Now consider my alternative. On Dr. Ro's Color Plate System you'll see three-quarters of your plate taken up with vegetables and fruit, beans, soy, and whole grains—the foods you usually think of as accompaniments to the main event—and only one-quarter of it covered with fish, chicken, turkey, or lean meat. This is a much healthier way to dress up a plate. But don't take my word for it: The American Institute for Cancer Research (AICR) recommends eating in this manner as a measure of cancer prevention. Why? Because this kind of meal plan emphasizes foods that are lower in calories and richer in antioxidants, phytochemicals, vitamins, and minerals, all of which help to ward off disease. According to the AICR, when combined with regular exercise, eating more plant foods and fewer animal foods can cut cancer rates by 40 percent. But it is not just for cancer prevention; it will also help prevent obesity, heart disease, diabetes, and the plethora of other chronic diseases and conditions that we've been suffering from for too long now.

What to Eat?

The reason we nutritionists are now more than ever recommending that you eat a variety of foods is because while much is known about what nutrients are in what foods and how those nutrients may help us, we still don't know nearly enough. So we're hedging our bets. Your best chance of getting the proper nutrients in the correct quantities is by eating a wide cross section of nutrient-rich foods. And calorie for calorie there is no better source of fiber and nutrients than plant foods. That is why I suggest 7–10 servings of fruits and vegetables, even though the Food Guide Pyramid encourages you to eat only 5–9 servings.

Don't get all wide-eyed. Eating this many fruits and vegetables is not only doable, it's easier than you may think. In the next secret, I'll show you how.

My Color Plate System teaches you to assemble a meal by thinking first about the color of your food, and then about the amounts and the proportions of food you put on your plate. It's a kind of quality control measure that helps to take the guesswork out of dining. Yet if you choose wisely, you get the benefit of optimal nutrition. Think of a lunch that mixes red, green,

Figure 9-1
Dr. Ro's Color Plate System Versus the Food Guide Pyramid

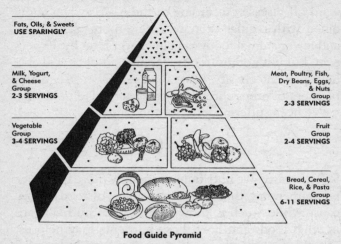

Food Guide Pyramid

Food Guide Pyramid	Dr. Ro's Color Plate System
Base includes 6–11 servings breads, cereals, rice, and pasta	Base contains 7–10 servings of fruits and vegetables
Next level includes 5–9 servings fruits and vegetables	3–4 total servings of protein foods (beans, nuts, soy, fish, chicken, turkey, lean red meat) and low-fat lactose-free or reduced-lactose dairy products
Next level includes 2–3 servings meat, fish, poultry, dry beans, eggs, and nuts; and 2–3 servings milk, yogurt, and cheese	3–4 servings of whole grains, including breads, cereal, and pasta
Next level includes fats, oils, and sugars, used sparingly	Modest amounts of oils and fats used with herbs and spices to flavor foods

and orange foods to protect against cancer. In other words, don't think of getting *over* the rainbow; ride that rainbow of colorful fruits and vegetables all the way to the promised land of good health!

What's in a Serving?

Since women require fewer calories than men do, I'll talk in terms of your needs as a sista. Not only are women confused about what to eat, but the question of how much is also baffling. Even when we sistas really want to lower our calories and fat intake, we don't always know how to go about doing it correctly, partly because we don't know what is meant by a serving size. One study pointed out that even nutritionists (the experts in the field) had trouble eyeballing food portions. Because of the giant portions served by the restaurant and fast-food industry, the question of what constitutes a "serving" has become so confusing in America that it's hard for anyone to tell anymore! So you find yourself wondering: Is that T-bone steak okay on your diet plan? Or is it so big that it wipes out a whole day's recommended intake? A good rule of thumb for a serving of meat, fish, or chicken is that it should look like the size of a makeup compact or a deck of cards. A serving of cooked vegetables looks like a half of a baseball. If you want to eyeball leafy raw veggies such as lettuce, think of a serving in terms of your fist. A serving of pasta or rice? Picture that same half baseball. And for a serving of dried cooked beans, you guessed it—the half baseball is the mental picture you want to have. But there are some more precise rules to follow, if you want to be exact. Take a look at the serving size guide that follows. Then try your hand at eyeballing what a serving of your food choices looks like and comparing your guesstimate with an actual measurement.

Degrees of Separation

There will be occasions when some of your menu items may be combination foods such as pasta dishes, beans and rice, or other kinds of casseroles, and you may not be sure how they fit into the color-plating system. Don't get hung up on details, which might cause you to get discouraged and just give up. Here are a few rules of thumb to follow in cases when the Color Plate System becomes a challenge.

* Always go for putting more vegetables and fruits on the plate and eating those before you get to the other part of the meal.
* When plating mixed dishes such as casseroles, beans and rice, pasta combinations, and so on, serve one cup of mixed dish to two cups of the vegetables, salad, and fruit. In other words, two-thirds of your plate is made up of fruits and vegetables.
* When serving a regular omelet or an egg-white omelet, think of it as protein food, covering one-third of your plate with the omelet and rounding out the plate with vegetables and/or fruit and a whole grain. You could also put

vegetables such as zucchini and mushrooms or a fruit such as tomatoes *in* the omelet.

❖ When preparing mixed dishes, always add veggies and/or fruits to the recipe when and where possible. A good example is a stir-fry, where you'd add a sprinkle of tofu, fish, chicken, or lean meat to vegetables such as broccoli, zucchini, or spinach. The veggie stir-fry would take up two-thirds of the plate, with the other third consisting of brown rice or whole-wheat pasta.

❖ When you are eating from a bowl, as in the case of cereal (hot oatmeal, cold soy cereal, etc.), add fresh fruit to the meal and consider it a done deal with those two dishes and a tall glass of water.

❖ Remember not to pile your plate to the ceiling. Part of the idea behind my Color Plate System is to eat foods that are better for you, but the rest involves controlling the portions of those foods.

Now that I've talked you into eating more fruits and vegetables, I want to give you some tips on buying, storing, and cooking them, so that you get the most out of their health potential.

Table 9-2 Serving Size Food Guide

Foods	Serving Size
Breads and cereals	1 slice bread 1 ounce ready-to-cook cereal $\frac{1}{2}$ cup cooked cereal, rice, or pasta
Vegetables	1 cup raw leafy vegetables $\frac{1}{2}$ cup cooked vegetables $\frac{1}{2}$ cup chopped raw vegetables $\frac{3}{4}$ cup vegetable juice
Soy products	Soybeans, $\frac{1}{2}$ cup Tofu, $\frac{1}{2}$ cup Prepared TVP, $\frac{1}{4}$ cup Soy cheese, 1 ounce Low-fat soy milk, 1 cup Roasted soy nuts, $\frac{1}{4}$ cup
Meats, fish, poultry	2–3 ounces cooked lean meat, poultry, or fish $\frac{1}{2}$ cup cooked dry beans 1 egg 4 egg whites 2 tablespoons peanut butter

Source: U.S. Department of Agriculture, Home and Garden Bulletin No. 252 (Washington, D.C.: USDA, 1992).

Organic Produce

With all of the talk about fresh produce, you might want to consider getting your fruits and vegetables without additions such as pesticides, hormones, and genetic manipulation. Don't get me wrong—not all pesticides are bad, nor is all genetically engineered produce bad, at least not in my opinion. Still, there may be reasons to purchase produce that has not been altered in any way and whose natural state has been preserved, and I know some of you feel strongly about such issues. Before October 2002 it was a veritable crapshoot as to whether or not it was even possible to be sure you were getting organic products. Now the USDA has issued government standards that apply to all products farmers produce and sell as "organic." These standards require them to ensure (by law) that all such products are in fact organically grown. And although a certain member of the U.S. Congress recently tried to undermine the standards that make "organic" a meaningful term, public outcry put an end to that attempt—at least for now.

Depending on the percentage of organic ingredients contained in a product, there are four different ways of classifying and labeling foods. Foods that are either 100 percent organic or 95–100 percent organic can bear a green seal that says "USDA Organic," and they are guaranteed to be free of hormones and antibiotics, irradiation, chemical- or sewer-based fertilizers, or any genetically modified organisms (GMOs). By the way, the USDA Organic label also pertains to animal products. They must have been treated humanely, not been given antibiotics or growth hormones, and fed organic feed. If a food is labeled "organic," which is the next classification, it must contain at least 70 percent organic ingredients. Finally, products containing less than 70 percent organic ingredients can list those ingredients and identify them as organic on the information panel on the side but cannot use the term "organic" anywhere on the front of the package, and also of course do not get to bear the organic seal.

Generally speaking, if you are uneasy about pesticides or GMOs, then it's worth it to buy organically produced foods, although you will pay more for them than you pay for their nonorganic counterparts. In my opinion, genetically modified foods have their place. You might prefer being able to bite into a juicy, red, sweet-tasting tomato rather than the often tasteless hothouse fruit you'd normally get at your corner grocery store. On the other hand, if your religion dictates that you not eat pork, then you might want to know that the genetic engineering that made it possible for the tomato to retain its natural juicy, sweet flavor and texture could involve the use of pork genes. The "organic" label guarantees that your food has not been genetically modified in such a fashion. The good news is that the government has now made it possible for the consumer to decide for herself whether she wants to spend that money.

Gaining Access to a High-Quality Food Supply

Okay, so you've got your shopping list loaded up with fruits and vegetables. Before you walk out the door, let's first talk about where the food is. You want the best possible food available for your family, yet your money is funny and you've got bills to pay. Even if you're a sista with a six-figure income, you may have other plans for your money. We all know that the more money you make, the more you need. And if I've heard it once, I've heard it a thousand times: "It costs a lot to eat good food." But I'm here to tell you this is not necessarily true.

Food Co-ops

A food co-op is a market where people buy food collectively in bulk, thus eliminating the middleman and cutting costs. There are probably food co-ops in your area; finding one may just take a little research. If there are no food co-ops nearby, and if you have an adventurous streak, the time may be right for you and your neighbors to join together and buy food in bulk for those in the group or extend the offer to other neighbors by selling it to them. A community room in the apartment complex you live in could serve as the space where you do business on the weekends, or maybe you could find space in a church basement or local community center.

In this scenario you and your partners decide on a day of the week to shop that fits the schedule of those involved, scout out the deals, and buy your food in bulk. This saves money, provides an opportunity for you and the other participants to control what you buy, and allows you (not the owner of the corner store) to control the quality of your food and the prices at which it is sold. Sometimes groups as small as half a dozen people join together in an effort like this. But groups like these have a way of growing, which is great because it allows you to rotate the work responsibilities among a greater number of people.

Farmer's Markets

Another option is the open-air farmer's market, where luscious produce is offered in abundance. Buying produce at a farmer's market often means getting the ripest produce available, produce that has often not been compromised by pesticides or preservatives. I consider this to be the next best option to growing the food myself. It is a chance to get back to nature, so to speak. Farmer's markets are available in the inner city, just as you would find them on the side of the road in rural America. In Washington, D.C., where I live, they exist in the 'hood. I frequent those, as well as roadside stands on the way to the country (in Virginia), where I spend summers and weekends. Here I find the ripest homegrown tomatoes and the freshest peaches and vegetables I've ever tasted. They are generally far superior to those I find in grocery stores.

Health Food Stores

In health food stores you will often find those obscure items that are not available in grocery store chains. Here there is a larger selection of unprocessed, unrefined foods. A large selection of soy products of all varieties is available here, although store chains such as Whole Foods Markets carry them, too. You will pay more for most foods in health food stores than you will pay for foods in traditional store chains, but if they are affordable, it's better to have the peace of mind.

Grocery Store Chains

I am happy to report that because the food industry has heard consumers who speak out about their food choices and food supply, many foods that were not available previously in food chains are there now. Take whole-wheat pasta, for example. It is on the store shelf at most major grocery chains now. But you must read the fine print on food labels for ingredients that you seek. Sometimes clever packaging, such as putting pasta made mostly from refined flour in a brown, "earthy"-looking box, could trick the consumer into thinking it's whole-wheat pasta. A closer look may reveal that it is in fact a combination of refined and whole-wheat flour in that pasta. Be careful and read, read, read. But by all means, go and ask for what you want. Your food dollar counts, and grocery store chains are listening.

Shopping Smarts

If you want to save money on food and buy those foods that are best for you, you'd better have a list. It's estimated that almost 50 percent of all food purchases are made on impulse. If want to capitalize on your food dollar, take heed:

❖ Keep a running list of your food needs by putting a piece of paper on the refrigerator to make a note of those staples that you need to replace as they run out. Get the family's input, but keep an eye on that list.

❖ Organize your grocery store list either by food group or by store layout. Whichever option you choose, don't leave home without the list!

❖ If organizing the list by store layout, make a note of the layout and make your list accordingly. If you get to the produce section of your store first, make produce the first group on your list.

❖ Keep an eye open for sales and specials at your favorite store chains. Clip coupons.

❖ Plan your shopping trips for twice a week. If you don't enjoy shopping, plan to buy staples once a month and perishables every two weeks.

❖ Check out a farmer's market or food co-op to get better-quality produce at better prices. Freeze the produce you don't need right away.

❖ Shop when you are not hungry and stick to that ever-loving list.

❖ Leave the kids at home or with a sitter when possible. They tend to encourage you to buy fattening treats.

❖ If you have a sweet tooth, buy snacks in small packages; this discourages you from eating the whole box in one sitting.

❖ Get the kids to help put away the groceries. This is a good exercise for them in what food is and how and where it is kept. It also saves you time.

Table 9-3 Produce Storage Guide

Vegetable	Storage Time
Asparagus	*Store in plastic bag in vegetable crisper compartment of fridge for up to 2 days*
Beets	*Store in fridge for 1 to 2 weeks*
Bell peppers	*Store in vegetable crisper for up to 3 to 5 days*
Broccoli	*Store in plastic zip-lock bags in vegetable crisper for up to 5 days*
Brussels sprouts	*Store in plastic bags in vegetable crisper for up to 5 days*
Cabbage	*Keep in vegetable crisper in fridge for up to 1 to 2 weeks*
Carrots	*Store in plastic bags in vegetable crisper for up to 1 to 2 weeks*
Cauliflower	*Store in vegetable crisper in fridge for up to 4 to 7 days*
Celery	*Store in vegetable crisper for up to 1 to 2 weeks*
Eggplant	*Store in plastic bag in fridge for up to 3 to 5 days*

Vegetable	Storage Time
Greens	*Store in plastic bag in fridge for 3 to 5 days*
Mushrooms	*Keep in original container or in paper bag (not in plastic bag) on fridge shelf (not crisper) for up to 3 days*
Okra	*Store in plastic bag in fridge for up to 5 days*
Onions	*Keep in cool, dry place (not near potatoes; onions will take on moisture of potatoes and decay quicker); do not store in fridge*
Potatoes	*Most potatoes will keep for up to 1½ months in a cool, dry place, away from sunlight*
Rutabagas	*Store in cool, dry, dark place for up to 2 months*
Salad greens (romaine and other lettuce, arugula, spinach, watercress)	*Rinse greens and dry; store between paper towels in fridge for up to 1 week*
String beans	*Store in plastic bags in vegetable crisper for up to 10 days*
Summer squash	*Store in fridge, unwashed in plastic bag, for up to 5 days*

Vegetable	Storage Time
Sweet potatoes	*Store in cool, dry place for up to 2 months*
Tomatoes	*Keep unwashed tomatoes at room temperature with the stems down, to preserve the flavor*
Turnips	*Keep in fridge, unwashed, in plastic bag for up to 1 week*
Winter squash	*Keep in cool, dry place for up to 2 months*

Produce Storage

Since most produce contains a heavy volume of water, it won't last long. When you buy fresh produce, you should generally plan to use it within three to four days, though some foods will keep longer. Beyond this period of time, rely on trusty frozen veggies and fruit; freezing does not compromise their nutritional value. Take a look at Table 9-3 for storage suggestions of commonly eaten vegetables.

Frequently Asked Questions

Q Dr. Ro: I've tried so hard to eat the number of fruits and vegetables you recommend, but it seems impossible to get in 7 to 10 servings a day. What am I doing wrong, and how will I ever get up to eating more?

A *I know your pain. I hear this all the time. Yet if you consider that a "real" serving of vegetables is a mere ½ cup and that a serving of fruit or vegetable juice is also just ½ cup, you might find it easy to do. Here are a few helpful hints to put you on track:*

❖ *Add vegetables to plain pizza.*

❖ *Add vegetables to salads, soups, stews, casseroles, and combination dishes such as spaghetti, lasagna, and sandwiches.*

❖ *Pack fruit in your bag and take it to work, school, the gym, or wherever you go. An apple, pear, orange, or banana is a great way to quell between-meal hunger pangs.*

❖ *Serve fruit for desserts in place of traditional favorites.*

❖ *Add fruit to cereals, salads, sandwiches, and side dishes to round out the perfect meal.*

❖ *Store cut veggies in plastic bags to keep on hand for snacks to munch on before and after workouts or while watching TV or doing work at your desk.*

Q **Dr. Ro: I've noticed a lot of snack foods made with vegetables. Are these a healthy way to eat more veggies to meet a more healthy goal?**

A *To meet the public demand for healthier foods, the food industry is responding to criticisms by developing foods like broccoli chips and other chips made with root vegetables. Just because a snack food claims to contain vegetables doesn't make it a health food. So listen up—and read the fine print. Ever seen Terra Chips? They're made with sliced sweet potato, yuca, taro root, and parsnip. But if you read the label, you find that they contain about 7 grams of fat per serving and only half the calcium of their traditional counterpart (tortilla chips), so you might as well opt for the Tostitos. Adding broccoli to the same old high-fat chips, even if the fats aren't trans fats, is no replacement for a serving of the real deal (broccoli). Your best bet is to cut those broccoli spears up and store them to eat as snacks, not substitute some cheap and fast imitation for good health. When you look a little closer, sometimes a "good thing" may not be as good as you think.*

Q **Dr. Ro: I like fruits and vegetables, but which ones are better for me as far as nutrition?**

A *I like a number of tropical fruits for their exotic flavor, but more important, they are packed with disease-fighting chemical compounds and nutrients that make them preferred favorites in many nutrition circles. My personal favorites, which I associate with an Afro-Caribbean menu, are:*

❖ *Mangoes, because they are rich in vitamins A and C, cancer-fighting beta-carotene, and fiber.*

❖ *Papayas, because they are loaded with vitamin C and carotenoids, are a great source of potassium and fiber, and have only about 55 calories per cup. Another plus is that they contain an enzyme that makes them handy in aiding digestion.*

❖ *Guavas, because they are rich in vitamins A and C, low in calories, and a good source of potassium.*

❖ *Pomegranates, because they are low-calorie, are rich in potassium and vitamin C, and contain antioxidants. Pomegranates, cultivated in tropical Africa, are a juicy red fruit with leathery skin whose real "meat" is found in sacks that encase tiny seeds. In the United States they range in color from deep orange to red. Scatter the seeds over a salad for a dish that is glowingly beautiful as well as nutritious.*

Some less exotic but very nutritious fruits that I enjoy include:

❖ *Persimmons, a rich orange-colored fruit. The large acorn-shaped Hachiya persimmons are meltingly sweet when they are soft and ripe, but quite unpleasant to eat until they are ripe. The smaller Fuyu persimmons, which look like small orange tomatoes, are tasty even when they are firm and crisp. Persimmons are rich in vitamins A and C, high in fiber, and a good source of potassium.*

❖ *Watermelon, which is low in calories and*

contains loads of vitamin C, carotenoids, and fiber.

✤ Oranges, because they contain plenty of fiber and are also a great source of vitamin C and folate. Eating a whole orange is far superior to drinking a glass of juice because the whole fruit is much higher in fiber.

✤ Grapefruit (pink or red), because it contains vitamin C, carotenoids, soluble fiber (which lowers cholesterol), and phytochemicals such as flavonoids, terpenes, and limonoids.

✤ Apricots, also rich in beta-carotene, potassium, and fiber. Canned and fresh apricots contribute some vitamin C to the diet, and although dried apricots have no vitamin C, they're a good source of iron.

Secret 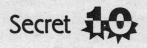 10

Dr. Ro's Plan to Kick-Start Your Way to Livin' Healthy: Menus, Recipes, and a Walking Workout

Vegetable Cookery

 So now that I've talked you into buying and eating more fruits and vegetables, what about cooking those vegetables to maximize their nutrition? In this secret, we'll cover that territory before going on to specific recipes. First, you should know that cooking your fresh vegetables should involve using as little water as possible to prevent leaching water-soluble vitamins such as vitamins C and B. Too much liquid means these nutrients end up in the water and not your body. It is good to use a vegetable steamer if you have one, but if not, just place a small amount of water in a nonstick pan, drop in the fresh veggies and seasoning (herbs and spices), and cover with a tight-fitting lid. Cook just until fork-tender for vegetables like broccoli or green beans, or until just wilted for greens, which may take only a few minutes for a green like spinach, or 30 minutes for greens like collards. Microwaving is another good way of cooking vegetables because it reduces both the amount of water they're cooked in and the time it takes to cook them, thus preserving valuable nutrients.

Seasoning for Your Colors

The days of pouring fat on top of good foods are long gone. You know too much now. There is a kind of responsibility that accompanies knowledge. Once you know something needs to be done, it's up to you to do it. So act on what you know, and season those good-for-you foods with additions that won't undo the health benefits you're trying to achieve.

If you're going to minimize your use of fat while maximizing tastiness, the first step is to learn a little about the difference between flavor enhancers and seasonings. When I ask a lot of my clients if they use seasonings to flavor foods, they always respond with a resounding yes. But when I delve a little deeper to find out just how they savor the flavor, I learn that they use salt. You see, they think salt is a seasoning. It is not. Once and for all, sistas, salt is a flavor enhancer. That means it brings out the existing flavor in food, but it does not add a different flavor. There's a reason I recommend seasonings over salt, and that is because salt raises blood pressure. Herbs, spices, and other seasonings do not.

How can we use seasonings to add flavor to this wonderful meal plan? Ever try squeezing a little lemon juice on broccoli? Or what about shaking a little cinnamon and nutmeg onto applesauce, oatmeal, or a sweet potato? Getting a little more exotic, how about adding a little curry powder and cayenne pepper to a broiled chicken breast? Girlfriend, that's what I call seasoning! Enough of this boring salt-and-pepper life! Curry powder, cinnamon, nutmeg, and cayenne pepper are all spices. They add liveliness to food well beyond the power of salt. There are thousands of spices, many brought from the motherland, the Caribbean, and the Orient, that will wake up the flavor in your food. You just need to know how to use them. Check out the suggestions that follow for a guide to putting the flavor back in your food.

Citrus

Use the juice, rind, and pulp of citrus fruits such as oranges, lemons, limes, and even pink grapefruits to add tanginess and bright color to vegetables, chicken, fish, and some soy dishes. Hint: Soy products like tofu take on the flavor of whatever you cook them in or put in or on them.

Spices

Cinnamon and nutmeg are good on baked fruits such as apples and bananas. Use ground, roasted, and whole spices such as cumin, allspice, curry powder, cinnamon, and crushed red pepper on meats, fish, poultry, soy, and vegetables. You can buy tasty spice rubs at any grocery store or have fun making up one of your own. One teaspoon paprika, one teaspoon dried oregano, and dashes of garlic powder, salt, cayenne, and Splenda make a tasty rub for meat. Massage it into the

Dr. Ro's Citrus Marinade for Chicken and Fish

1/4 cup olive oil

2 tablespoons balsamic vinegar

2 tablespoons fresh lime juice

1/2 tablespoon minced ginger

1 tablespoon chopped fresh parsley

1 tablespoon chopped fresh thyme

With a wire whisk, blend the ingredients together in a small bowl. Marinate chicken or fish in a covered dish for 3 to 4 hours in the fridge. ■

Dr. Ro's Citrus Marinade for Meat and Soy

1/3 cup blackstrap molasses

1/4 cup orange juice

1/3 cup prepared Dijon mustard

1/3 cup balsamic vinegar

3 tablespoons Worcestershire sauce

1 teaspoon hot sauce or Tabasco sauce

Combine the ingredients in a small bowl and use for grilling, broiling, or basting any meat or meat substitute, such as tofu products. ■

meat and let it sit for an hour or two before cooking. For an Indian flavor, try combining cumin, cloves, cinnamon, coriander, and a dash of cayenne—a great rub for chicken breast or a fatty fish like salmon. You could also make up a dried herb mixture, my personal favorite, by mixing dried tarragon, thyme, basil, and parsley; be sure to add garlic powder and peppercorns for a lively tasty flavor for meat, chicken, or fish. If you want to make enough for several meals, blend all of these ingredients together, removing stems and seeds, and store in a small container with a tight-fitting lid in a cool, dry place. Don't be afraid to try new and different things. Experiment and find what works best for your taste buds.

Chili Peppers

Chilis are a spicy addition to any dish. Put them in tomato sauces, or just use them to add excitement to any dish that's missing that "something special." Experiment with different kinds of peppers, like jalapeños, which vary from mild to medium hot; serranos, which are mainly hot; poblanos, an all-purpose pepper of varying hotness; or even habaneros (but tread lightly with these), small, usually orange peppers that have a very complex flavor and a reputation for being the hottest pepper in the world. Habaneros are often confused with Scotch bonnets, a pepper widely used throughout the Caribbean and a possible contender for the title of hottest pepper.

Mustard

Try mustard seeds or Dijon mustard in almost anything, from tuna to potatoes to balsamic vinaigrette dressing. There are no calories to consider with mustard, and the tang it adds to these dishes makes them something special. There are also herb-flavored mustards (like tarragon) and hot and spicy mustard, which can be great in dressings, sauces, marinades, and sandwiches.

Soy Sauce and Teriyaki

If you want to add flavor to Asian-inspired meals, soy dishes, and noodle entrées, get out the soy and teriyaki sauces. They both make great marinades, too. But be sure to buy the low-sodium version of these products, because otherwise the sodium content is through the roof.

Vegetables

I can't say it enough: Vegetables are the root of a great diet. But their use in flavoring other vegetable dishes and entrées is underestimated. Sure, you're used to putting sliced onions on a steak, but what about topping a baked potato or a healthy serving of greens or green beans with chopped spring onions? Or what about adding tomatoes and carrots to a big old pot of beans? Ever thought about adding celery to a green salad? It's not just for potato salad or egg salad. Add celery to a salad, throw in some walnuts and apple slices or orange sections, toss with a dressing made of low-fat plain yogurt, a dash of Dijon mustard, and a pinch of curry powder or ground cumin, and you've got the makings of a dish that can serve as a main course for lunch or a light dinner. Use your imagination and be creative!

Herbology

Herbs add not just flavor but substance to your diet. Take parsley, for example. It contains rich amounts of vitamins A and C, which help protect against cancer. Parlsey also contains more histidine, an amino acid that aids in the prevention of tumors, than most vegetables. Furthermore, parsley is a great source of potassium, which helps to lower blood pressure, and of folic acid, the B vitamin that helps prevent birth defects and may combat heart disease. Sage, on the other hand, mostly known in our community for its contribution to stuffing and chicken dishes, contains flavonoids, which have estrogen-like effects that calm night sweats and hot flashes and protect against heart disease, too. These are just two examples of how far herbs can go to make you healthy while providing great taste and texture to the perfect meal. But that's not all. Some herbs are believed to have a calming effect on the body and the spirit.

I prefer to use fresh herbs to season food, but on occasion I use dried herbs, too. You can buy fresh herbs in the produce section of most grocery store chains, but growing them is easy. My uncle and I plant an herb garden in the country, where my mom grew up, every summer. I keep a few herbs, peppers, and tomatoes in my backyard in the city, too—you can even grow them in pots on the windowsill if you don't have a yard or garden. Whether you decide to try your green thumb at growing your own herbs or shop in the produce section, hang them upside down to air-dry to preserve whatever you don't use immediately. Once dried, store them in airtight jars or zip-lock bags, then simply toss them into your favorite recipes when the time comes.

After making the case for seasoning with herbs and spices, I would be remiss if I didn't give you a reference for how to use them. Take a look at the following chart to get great ideas for how to season your color plates with wonderful, aromatic flavors that won't disappoint. Copy this chart and pin it on your fridge for at-your-fingertips hints to use in the kitchen.

Table 10-1 Herb and Spice Food Compatibility

Herb	Compatible Foods
Allspice	*Fruit dishes, sweet potatoes*
Basil	*Fish, spaghetti, tomatoes, sauces, poultry; great in pesto*
Celery seed	*Potato salad, soups, stuffing*
Cilantro (fresh)	*Lemony-tasting leaves; great in salsas, soups, sauces, eggs, sandwiches, Thai dishes*
Cinnamon	*Mild, sweet flavor; brings out the flavor of chicken; great in apple dishes and oatmeal*

Herb	Compatible Foods
Cloves	*Keen, sharp taste; great in low-fat pork cuts (such as pork tenderloin), teas, and Caribbean dishes*
Coriander (seeds)	*Nutty, aromatic seeds; good in fruity dishes, especially bananas, apples, pears, peaches, and pomegranates; also makes aromatic rice*
Cumin	*Another seed with an aromatic, nutty taste; great with anything curried*
Dill weed	*Similar to the aroma of caraway; good with cabbage, salmon, and other fish, dips made with yogurt*
Garlic	*Perfect for almost anything; all vegetable, chicken, meat, and soy dishes*
Ginger root	*Great in teas, curries, chicken, apple, and other fruit dishes*
Lemongrass	*An Asian favorite with a tremendously soothing aroma; great in teas, rice, Thai dishes*
Mint	*Great in teas, chicken, salads, fruit dishes*
Nutmeg	*Warm, spicy, and sweet; no baked sweet potato is complete without it; also good in fruit dishes, salads, chicken, and squash*
Oregano	*Peppery, spicy leaves; an Italian favorite used with fish, chicken, pasta, tomatoes*

Herb	Compatible Foods
Paprika	*A mild to hot peppery powder; don't dare put potato salad, deviled eggs, or mac and cheese on a black person's table without this one; also good on whole grains, beans, and pastas*
Parsley	*Slightly peppery but mild, fresh taste; a great garnish for almost anything (not a bad breath freshener, either); makes good tea, but also good as a complement to potatoes, fish, poultry, pasta, vegetables*
Rosemary	*Aromatic sprigs with just a hint of lemon and pine; great in any Italian dish, chicken and poultry, stuffing, egg whites, baked fruit dishes*
Sage	*Slightly bitter leaves; you can't do chicken, turkey, or stuffing without sage; also great with veal, potatoes, squash, onions, other vegetables, pasta, beans*
Spring onions	*Pungent odor and flavor; another West Indian favorite; great with meats, poultry, fish, vegetables, egg whites, salads; a staple in any homemade herbal mix*
Tarragon	*Greenish flowery herb with a licorice taste; great in soups, stews; I love it on chicken, salmon, meats, vegetables*
Thyme	*A West Indian favorite with a lemony aroma; wakes up the flava in chicken, fish, meats, vegetables; blends well with garlic, basil, curry*

Kick-Start Your Way to
Livin' Healthy with Food

The menus that accompany this meal plan are based on an average of 1,500 to 2,000 calories a day. Why so low, you ask? Mostly because it is well established in this book and elsewhere that we eat too much food. It is this caloric excess that is digging us into early graves. By now you should have calculated your energy needs, so adjust your calorie level to the one that fits you individually. The average sedentary woman who is five feet five inches tall will probably not require much more food than this. If you need to lose weight, adjust your calorie level by subtracting 500 calories per day. Increase your activity level and change your routine periodically as you settle into an exercise regimen. We'll talk about that later, but first—the food.

Sample Menus to Kick-Start
Your Way to Livin' Healthy

Day 1

Breakfast
$1/2$ cup whole-grain cereal with soy protein
1 cup nonfat lactose-free milk (if lactose-intolerant);
   any nonfat milk, including soy milk, will work
1 cup blueberries
8 ounces water

Midmorning snack
Dr. Ro's Soy-Fruity Shake
   (made with berries, citrus, bananas, and
   soy powder with genisten)
16 ounces water

Lunch
Dr. Ro's Black Bean Hoppin' John
   ($1/2$ cup Dr. Ro's Black Beans with $1/2$ cup Dr. Ro's
   Brown Rice Medley)
Ro's Bell-Ringin' Spinach Salad with balsamic
   vinaigrette
8 ounces tomato juice
8 ounces water

Midday Snack

1 small banana

16 ounces water

Dinner

4 ounces Dr. Ro's North Carolina Barbecue That
   Gobbles (vinegar-based pulled turkey barbecue)

1 ear yellow corn on the cob (steamed or grilled),
   fat-free butter-flavor sprinkles (optional)

2 cups steamed broccoli, carrots, and tomato,
   seasoned with fresh cilantro and basil

1 cup sliced watermelon

16 ounces herbal tea with fresh mint leaves (sugar
   substitute optional)

Evening Snack

8 ounces orange juice

6 graham crackers made with whole-wheat flour

Nutritional Analysis: *calories: 1,755, protein: 92.9 grams,
carbohydrate: 330 grams, fat: 21 grams, cholesterol: 55.6
milligrams, vitamin A: 45,057 IU, vitamin C: 855 milligrams, dietary fiber: 82.2 grams*

Day 2

Breakfast
1 cup cooked oatmeal with raisins, cinnamon,
and a sprinkle of brown sugar
1 cup soy milk
6 ounces fresh orange juice
8 ounces water

Midmorning Snack
1 cup fresh blueberries
8 ounces water

Lunch
Turkey burger on whole-wheat bun with lettuce,
tomato, onion, alfalfa sprouts, and reduced-fat
mayo
Dr. Ro's Bell-Ringin' Spinach Salad
6 ounces fresh orange juice

Midday Snack
1 medium apple
16 ounces water

Dinner
Dr. Ro's Seafood-Tofu Stir-Fry
Mixed green salad with vinaigrette dressing
1 cup fresh pineapple, cubed
16 ounces iced ginger tea made with fresh ginger
boiled in water, cooled (sugar substitute optional)
8 ounces water

Evening Snack

> 1 handful (about 28) dry-roasted peanuts
> 8 ounces fruit punch made from a combination of
>   100 percent fruit juices

Nutritional Analysis: *calories: 1,801, protein: 73.3 grams, carbohydrate: 255 grams, fat: 62.6 grams, saturated fat: 8.7 grams, cholesterol: 91 milligrams, vitamin A: 11,403 IU, vitamin C: 429.5 milligrams, dietary fiber: 34.1 grams*

Day 3

Breakfast

> Egg-white omelet made with 3 egg whites, ¼ cup
>   chopped red bell peppers, ¼ cup chopped green
>   bell peppers, and ¼ small onion, chopped
> 1 slice whole-wheat toast with marmalade
> 8 ounces apple juice

Midmorning snack

> 1 cup raw carrots
> ½ cup broccoli florets
> 8 ounces water

Lunch

> Tuna sandwich on whole-wheat pita bread with
>   lettuce, tomato, and reduced-fat mayo
> 1 cup tomato soup
> ½ mango
> 16 ounces water

Midday Snack

12 ounces Dr. Ro's Soy-Fruity Shake
8 ounces water

Dinner

Dr. Ro's N'awlins Butter Beans with
    Chicken Andouille Sausage
Dr. Ro's Corny Bread
Green salad with vinaigrette dressing
6 ounces fruit juice, chilled
1/2 cup fresh berries

Evening Snack

1 ounce dry-roasted soy nuts
8 ounces water

Nutritional Analysis: *calories: 1,578, protein: 77.7 grams, carbohydrate: 262.7 grams, fat: 30 grams, cholesterol: 59 milligrams, vitamin A: 46,280 IU, vitamin C: 331 milligrams, dietary fiber: 24.7 grams*

Day 4

Breakfast

1/2 cup whole-grain cereal with soy protein
1 cup nonfat lactose-free milk (or any nonfat milk)
1 cup strawberries
16 ounces water
1 cup ginger tea with sugar substitute (optional)

Midmorning Snack

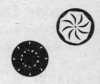

1 small apple
1 ounce low-fat cheese
6 whole-wheat crackers
8 ounces water

Lunch

Turkey sandwich with 3 ounces fresh sliced turkey on
    whole-grain bread with Dijon mustard, lettuce,
    and sprouts
Dr. Ro's Tricolor Pepper Salad
1 cup white grapes
16 ounces iced herbal tea with sugar substitute
    (optional)

Midday Snack

1 ostrich stick, teriyaki or barbecue flavor (tastes like a
    Slim Jim, only has 1 gram of fat and 10 grams of
    protein)
16 ounces water

Dinner

Dr. Ro's Citrus Barbecued Salmon
Sautéed spinach in olive oil with garlic
    and fresh mushrooms
Fresh sliced tomatoes with balsamic vinegar
8 ounces limeade made with fresh lime juice, sugar
    substitute (optional), and water topped with
    mint leaves

Evening Snack
$1/2$ cup raw carrots
8 ounces water

Nutritional Analysis: *calories: 1,526, protein: 90.8 grams, carbohydrate: 245 grams, fat: 29.5 grams, saturated fat: 4.8 grams, cholesterol: 97 milligrams, vitamin A: 23,695 IU, vitamin C: 425 milligrams, calcium: 916 milligrams, dietary fiber: 33 grams*

Day 5

Breakfast
$1/2$ cup soy protein cereal with $1/2$ cup nonfat
    lactose-free milk (or any nonfat milk)
$1/2$ cup fresh strawberries
6 ounces fresh orange juice
16 ounces water

Midmorning Snack
12 ounces Dr. Ro's Soy-Fruity Shake with pineapple
    juice, bananas, and soy powder with genisten
16 ounces water

Lunch
1 cup Big Mama's Smoked Turkey-Barley Soup
6 whole-wheat crackers
8 ounces fruit punch made with a
    mixture of 100 percent fruit juices
16 ounces water

Midday Snack

1 medium banana
16 ounces water

Dinner

3 ounces rotisserie chicken breast
1/2 cup steamed mixed vegetables with fresh herbs
1 medium vine-ripened tomato, sliced, with balsamic
vinegar
1/2 cup steamed brown rice medley
1 cup citrus sections with fresh mint
16 ounces water

Evening Snack

1 pomegranate
8 ounces water

Nutritional Analysis: *calories: 1,571, protein: 70 grams, carbohydrate: 290 grams, fat: 19.8 grams, saturated fat: 4.6 grams, cholesterol: 83.9 milligrams, calcium: 1,265 milligrams, vitamin C: 376 milligrams, dietary fiber: 24 grams*

Day 6

Breakfast

1/2 cup oatmeal with 1/2 cup soy milk, cinnamon, and
1 teaspoon raisins
1 slice whole-wheat toast with 1 teaspoon apple butter
1 cup ginger tea with sugar substitute (optional)
8 ounces water

Midmorning Snack

  $^{1}/_{2}$ cup canned plums
  16 ounces water
  1 cup plain fat-free yogurt

Lunch

  1 cup Dr. Ro's Mixed-Grain Pilaf
  1 cup tomato soup
  6 whole-wheat crackers
  $^{1}/_{2}$ cup raw carrots
  16 ounces water

Midday Snack

  1 medium apple
  1 tablespoon peanut butter
  6 whole-wheat crackers
  16 ounces water

Dinner

  2 ounces Dr. Ro's Ire Snapper Fillets
  $^{1}/_{2}$ cup Dr. Ro's Country-City Cabbage with fresh dill
  $^{1}/_{2}$ cup steamed carrots
  1 cup vegetable juice
  8 ounces water

Evening Snack

  1 cup air-popped popcorn with fat-free
     butter-flavored sprinkles
  1 cup grape juice
  16 ounces water

Nutritional Analysis: *calories: 1,634, protein: 60.5 grams, carbohydrate: 285 grams, fat: 33 grams, saturated fat: 7.9* grams, cholesterol: 53 milligrams, calcium: 1,224 milligrams, vitamin C: 209 milligrams, dietary fiber: 29.7 grams

Day 7

Breakfast

$\frac{1}{2}$ cup Dr. Ro's Steamed Rainbow Potatoes and
Onions
$\frac{1}{2}$ cup Dr. Ro's Country Steamed Apples
with a Twist
3 strips of broiled turkey bacon
$\frac{1}{2}$ cup strawberries and blueberries, mixed
6 ounces orange juice
8 ounces water

Midmorning Snack

$\frac{1}{2}$ cup soy cereal
1 fresh peach
16 ounces water

Lunch

1 cup Dr. Ro's New-Soul Mac-n-Cheese
1 broiled tomato
Mixed green salad with balsamic vinaigrette
16 ounces water

Midday Snack

28 roasted peanuts in the shell
16 ounces water

Dinner

4 ounces Dr. Ro's New-Soul Turkey Meatloaf
½ cup Dr. Ro's Baked Sweet Potatoes with
    Apples-n-Raisins
½ cup Dr. Ro's Lean Greens
6 ounces orange juice
8 ounces water

Evening Snack

1 medium nectarine
8 ounces water

Nutritional Analysis: *calories: 2,015, protein: 51.5 grams, carbohydrate: 378 grams, fat: 40 grams, cholesterol: 56 milligrams, saturated fat: 6.5 grams, vitamin C: 377 milligrams, calcium: 1,032 milligrams, vitamin A: 22,099 IU, dietary fiber: 42 grams*

Sample Recipes to Kick-Start
Your Way to Livin' Healthy

The recipes I've included come from a rich Afro-Caribbean tradition of black people whose paths I've crossed, whether from my own Virginia family or from the many colleagues, friends, and mentors I've encountered along the way. Here you'll get some of my mama's recipes and those of her mama and her family (anything that refers to "country" comes from my family). But there are other recipes for truly good food that were spawned from other southern roots, such as those of my guardian, Rosetta, who was from Rocky Mount, North Carolina. There they do barbecue a certain way, different from that found in Texas or any other part of the country. If there is one thing I've learned, don't mess with black folks' 'cue. I've made a few changes to give it a healthful twist; still, it has the flava black folks have come to love. You will also find recipes that have maintained their rich heritage from the motherland but made the trek to us here by way of the Caribbean. Try the Ire Red Snapper; I know you'll love it.

If ever you want to know how similar, rather than different, people are, just look at the food. Think of Jollof Rice from Senegal (nothing more than black-eyed peas and rice), known as Hoppin' John in North Carolina and other parts of the South. I call my own creation Black Bean Hoppin' John, and it makes for an interesting and nutritious combination.

Use these recipes, then add your own flava to satisfy your family's palate. But at all costs, maintain the healthy premise on which these recipes are based. Remember, the goal is to have the foods you love. Try a few new foods along the way, and do it all in the interest of taking care of you and yours. Enjoy!

Dr. Ro's Citrus Barbecued Salmon

▼▼▼▼▼

$1/4$ orange juice concentrate

$1/2$ cup lime juice concentrate

$1/2$ cup barbecue sauce

1 pound salmon fillet

2 tablespoons fresh thyme, dill, and rosemary, combined

Salt and freshly ground pepper to taste

Olive oil cooking spray

$1/2$ lemon, thinly sliced

Few sprigs of fresh dill

Mix the juice concentrates and barbecue sauce together in a small bowl and set aside.

Rub the fish with the fresh herbs and salt and pepper on both sides. Spray a nonstick grill pan or large nonstick skillet with the olive oil spray and heat the pan. Sear the fish in the hot pan until brown on both sides. The fish is done when it flakes with a fork (about 10 minutes). Coat the fish with the citrus-barbecue sauce mixture and heat, then remove from the pan. Twist the lemon slices to curl, then place on top of the fish with the dill sprigs as a garnish. Serves 4.

Nutritional Analysis: *calories/serving: 183, protein: 23 grams, carbohydrate: 14 grams, fat: 4 grams, saturated fat: 0.7 grams, cholesterol: 58 milligrams, dietary fiber: 1.1 grams, vitamin C: 27 milligrams* ■

Dr. Ro's New-Soul Turkey Meatloaf

Olive oil cooking spray

2 egg whites

½ pound ground turkey

½ pound firm tofu

½ cup oatmeal

1 cup chopped onion

½ cup chopped green and red
bell pepper, combined

½ cup tomato juice

1 tablespoon Worcestershire
sauce

1 teaspoon salt

½ teaspoon freshly ground
black pepper

½ cup tomato sauce

*P*reheat the oven to 350°F. Lightly spray a 9½ × 5½ × 3½-inch nonstick loaf pan or a glass baking dish with olive oil cooking spray.

Beat the egg whites in a small bowl. Blend with all the remaining ingredients, except the ½ cup tomato sauce. Form the meatloaf into the shape of a loaf and place in the nonstick baking pan. Spread the tomato sauce over the meatloaf and bake, uncovered, for 1 hour and 15 minutes. Let stand for 5 minutes before serving. Serves 6.

Nutritional Analysis: *calories/serving: 171, protein: 14.5 grams, carbohydrate: 14.7 grams, fat: 6.4 grams, saturated fat: 1.4 grams, cholesterol: 33.6 milligrams, dietary fiber: 2.4 grams, vitamin C: 13.8 milligrams* ■

Dr. Ro's Lean Greens

2 bunches of greens (collards, kale, mustard, or turnip)

1 tablespoon olive oil

1½ cups defatted chicken or vegetable broth

¼ cup water

½ cup finely chopped spring onions

½ teaspoon minced garlic

⅛ teaspoon salt (optional)

⅛ teaspoon cayenne pepper

¼ teaspoon chopped fresh thyme

¼ teaspoon chopped fresh basil

¼ teaspoon liquid smoke (optional, if you like smoked greens)

Cut the greens into strips. Add the oil to a large pan, then sauté the greens until wilted, tender, and bright green. Add the broth, ¼ cup water, and the remaining ingredients. Simmer for approximately 15–30 minutes. The greens should be firm, tender, and bright green, preserving nutrients, flavor, and texture. Serves 2.

Nutritional Analysis: *calories: 58, cholesterol: 0, fat: approx. 5 grams, sodium: 182 milligrams* ■

Dr. Ro's Savory Black Beans
(for Black Bean Hoppin' John)

½ cup chopped carrot

Olive oil cooking spray

1 16-ounce can black beans

2 tablespoons blackstrap
    molasses

2 tablespoons brown sugar

⅛ teaspoon crushed garlic

½ cup chopped red onion

*I*n a small pan, sauté the chopped carrot in olive oil cooking spray until tender. In another pan, heat the beans with the molasses, brown sugar, garlic, and cooked carrot. Serve the beans topped with the chopped red onion. Serves 4 to 6.

Nutritional Analysis: *calories: 142, protein: 6.3 grams, carbohydrate: 26.7 grams, fat: 0.9 grams, cholesterol: 0 milligrams, dietary fiber: 6.5 grams, vitamin A: 2,134 IU* ■

Dr. Ro's Brown Rice Medley

2 cups quick-cooking
   brown rice
½ cup chopped fresh
   mushrooms

· 1 teaspoon salt
Freshly ground pepper
   to taste

*B*oil the rice as directed on the package. Add the mushrooms to the rice 5 minutes before the rice is completely cooked. Add salt and pepper to taste. Serve with Black Bean Hoppin' John or any other entrée you desire. Serves 4.

Nutritional Analysis: *calories: 115, protein: 2.6 grams, carbohydrate: 24 grams, fat: 0.9 grams, saturated fat: 0.18 grams, cholesterol: 0 milligrams* ■

Dr. Ro's North Carolina Barbecue
That Gobbles

2 pounds smoked turkey
   (breast mixed with
   drumsticks)
½ teaspoon seasoned salt
1 small onion, chopped
2 teaspoons olive oil

1 tablespoon crushed
   red pepper
½ teaspoon cayenne pepper
1 cup apple cider vinegar
1 tablespoon crushed garlic

*I*n a large pot, boil the smoked turkey parts with the seasoned salt and enough water to cover until tender (about 1½ hours—the meat should fall off the bone). When the meat is cool, pull the meat from the bones and separate it into small pieces (the meat should be fairly stringy) and set aside. In a large pan, sauté the onion in olive oil until tender. Add the crushed red pepper, cayenne pepper, vinegar, garlic, and meat to the onion and simmer over low heat until the ingredients are fully blended. Serve with greens and corn-on-the-cob, or make barbecue sandwiches on whole-wheat buns. Serves 4.

Nutritional Analysis: *calories: 175, protein: 30.2 grams, carbohydrate: 0.3 grams, fat: 6.2 grams, saturated fat: 0.6 grams, cholesterol: 66.9 milligrams, dietary fiber: 0 grams* ∎

Dr. Ro's Wilted Granny Smith Spinach Salad with Apple Cider Vinaigrette

2 pounds fresh spinach, washed

2 medium Granny Smith apples, washed and cored

½ cup lemon juice

Apple Cider Vinaigrette (recipe follows)

1 cup chopped walnuts

*P*lace the cleaned spinach in a colander to drain, then transfer the spinach to a large nonstick sauté pan and heat until the spinach becomes bright green (about 1 to 2 minutes), but firm and slightly limp. Slice the apples evenly and thinly, leaving the skins on. In a bowl, place the apple slices in the lemon juice. (Note: Lemon juice prevents apples from turning brown and keeps them crisp.) Toss the spinach with the sliced apples, then pour the vinaigrette over the salad and toss. Sprinkle the chopped nuts over the salad and serve warm. Serves 4.

Nutritional Analysis: *calories: 119, protein: 3.8 grams, carbohydrate: 18.3 grams, fat: 4.4 grams, saturated fat: 0.5 grams, cholesterol: 0 milligrams, calcium: 98 milligrams, vitamin A: 5,921 IU, dietary fiber: 4.4 grams* ■

Apple Cider Vinaigrette

½ cup apple cider vinegar

½ cup apple cider

1 tablespoon brown sugar

1 teaspoon ground allspice

1 teaspoon olive oil

In a small bowl, blend the vinegar, cider, brown sugar, allspice, and olive oil to a smooth consistency and set aside.

Nutritional Analysis: *calories: 27.9, protein: 0 grams, carbohydrate: 2.8 grams, fat: 1.2 grams, saturated fat: 1.2 grams, cholesterol: 0 milligrams, dietary fiber: 0 grams* ■

Dr. Ro's Bell-Ringin' Spinach Salad with Strawberries and Raspberry Vinaigrette

2 pounds fresh spinach

1 cup fresh strawberries, halved

1 cup sliced red bell peppers

Raspberry Vinaigrette (recipe follows)

¼ cup fresh raspberries

Wash the spinach and drain in a colander. Place the spinach in a large salad bowl and add ¾ of the strawberries and the peppers. Pour the vinaigrette over the salad and toss. Sprinkle with the remaining fruit. Serves 4.

Nutritional Analysis: *calories: 32, protein: 3.7 grams, carbohydrate: 5 grams, fat: 0.5 grams, saturated fat: 0 grams, cholesterol: 0 milligrams, vitamin A: 8,122 IU, vitamin C: 118 milligrams, calcium: 97 milligrams, dietary fiber: 11.4 grams* ∎

Raspberry Vinaigrette

½ cup raspberry juice   ½ cup balsamic vinegar
  concentrate
¼ cup fresh raspberries

In a small bowl, blend the raspberry juice concentrate, the fresh raspberries, and balsamic vinegar and mash to a slightly smooth consistency. Set aside.

Nutritional Analysis: *calories: 17.5, protein: 0.1 grams, carbohydrate: 3.8 grams, fat: 0 grams, saturated fat: 0 grams, dietary fiber: 1 gram* ∎

Big Mama's Smoked Turkey-Barley Soup

Olive oil cooking spray

1½ pounds smoked turkey drumsticks, cooked and cut into small pieces

2 10-ounce cans defatted chicken broth or fat-free vegetable broth

1 cup water

1 cup coarsely chopped green cabbage

1 cup coarsely chopped red cabbage

1 cup chopped carrot

1 cup chopped onion

1 cup chopped peeled rutabaga

⅓ cup quick-cooking barley

1 teaspoon chopped fresh thyme or ½ teaspoon dried thyme

1 teaspoon chopped fresh rosemary or ½ teaspoon dried rosemary

½ teaspoon crushed garlic

½ teaspoon ground allspice

½ teaspoon freshly ground black pepper

1 bay leaf

*L*ightly spray a Dutch oven with olive oil cooking spray. Heat the pan over medium heat until it is hot. Add the cooked smoked turkey pieces and sauté until browned, about 5 minutes. Add the broth, water, and the remaining ingredients; bring to a boil. Cover and reduce the heat. Simmer for 25 minutes, or until the meat and barley are tender. Be sure to stir occasionally. Discard the bay leaf. Serves 4.

Nutritional Analysis: *calories: 182, protein: 20 grams, carbohydrate: 13.1 grams, fat: 5.1 grams, saturated fat: 1.7 grams, cholesterol: 52 milligrams, vitamin A: 5,719 IU, dietary fiber: 2.7 grams* ∎

Dr. Ro's Mixed Grain Pilaf

½ cup cooked quinoa
  (see Note)

½ cup cooked kasha

Olive oil cooking spray

½ cup thinly sliced fresh
  mushrooms

½ cup chopped onions

4 spring (green) onions,
  chopped

½ cup sliced celery

1 teaspoon crushed garlic

2 cups defatted chicken broth

½ teaspoon chopped fresh
  rosemary

½ teaspoon salt

½ teaspoon ground white
  pepper

*C*ook grains according to package instructions, then set aside. Spray a heavy nonstick skillet with cooking spray. Add the mushrooms, onions, celery, and garlic and sauté until tender but firm. Add the grains. Slowly stir in the broth, rosemary, and the salt and pepper. Bring to a boil over high heat, reduce the heat, cover, and simmer for 20 minutes, or until the liquid is absorbed and the grains and vegetables are chewy. Makes 4 small (⅓-cup) servings.

Note: Before quinoa (pronounced keen-WA) is cooked, to remove its bitter taste it should be washed in a colander under running water until the water runs clear.

Nutritional Analysis: *calories: 141, protein: 6.7 grams, carbohydrate: 24.8 grams, fat: 1.9 grams, saturated fat: 0.2 grams, cholesterol: 0 milligrams, vitamin A: 2,945 IU, vitamin C: 18 milligrams, dietary fiber: 2.5 grams* ■

Dr. Ro's Tricolor Pepper Salad

Balsamic Vinaigrette
  (recipe follows)

1 cup chopped
  red bell pepper

1 cup chopped
  green bell pepper

1 cup chopped
  yellow bell pepper

1 pound mixed salad greens
  (spring mix): arugula,
  spinach, romaine lettuce,
  green leaf lettuce

Marinate the peppers in half the vinaigrette for 45 minutes. Wash the salad greens and drain in a colander. Toss the salad greens in the remaining vinaigrette dressing. Spoon the marinated pepper mixture over the salad greens and serve chilled. Serves 4 to 6.

Nutritional Analysis: calories: 137, protein: 1.5 grams, carbohydrate: 16.3 grams, fat: 7.4 grams, saturated fat: 1 gram, cholesterol: 0 milligrams, vitamin A: 5,455 IU, vitamin C: 172.7 milligrams, dietary fiber: 2.4 grams ■

Balsamic Vinaigrette

4 teaspoons Dijon mustard

½ cup balsamic vinegar

4 tablespoons olive oil

2 teaspoons sugar substitute

Combine the vinaigrette ingredients in a small bowl.

Dr. Ro's Baked Sweet Potatoes
with Apples-n-Raisins

▚▚▚▚

4 medium sweet potatoes,
   unpeeled

Butter-flavored vegetable oil
   cooking spray

1 medium Granny Smith
   apple, unpeeled, cored,
   quartered, and sliced

1 medium McIntosh apple,
   unpeeled, cored, quartered,
   and sliced

½ cup seedless raisins

½ teaspoon each cinnamon,
   nutmeg, allspice, combined

½ cup apple juice or apple
   cider

1 tablespoon blackstrap
   molasses

1 teaspoon reduced-fat
   margarine

*B*oil the potatoes until tender, roughly 30 minutes. Remove the
skins and discard. Slice the potatoes.

Preheat the oven to 425°F. Lightly spray a 1-quart baking dish
with cooking spray.

Layer the potatoes with the apples and raisins. In a small mixing bowl, blend the spice mixture and juice, then heat the mixture
in a small saucepan until smooth. Pour over the potato layers.
Drizzle the molasses on top of the potatoes. Dot with the margarine, sprinkle a smidgen of cinnamon and nutmeg over the top,
and bake, uncovered, 20 minutes, or until bubbly and thoroughly
heated. Serves 6.

Nutritional Analysis: *calories: 174, protein: 1.9 grams, carbohydrate: 41 grams, fat: 1 gram, saturated fat: 0.2 grams, cholesterol:*

0 milligrams, vitamin A: 17,482 IU, vitamin C: 22.9 milligrams, dietary fiber: 4.3 grams ■

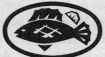

Dr. Ro's Ire Snapper Fillets

2 pounds red snapper fillets (about 6 fillets)

1 red bell pepper, sliced and cut into strips

1 green bell pepper, sliced and cut into strips

1 yellow bell pepper, sliced and cut into strips

1 orange bell pepper, sliced and cut into strips

1 medium onion, peeled, sliced, and cut into strips

4 to 6 spring onions, chopped

2 tablespoons crushed garlic

1 tablespoon olive oil

Olive oil cooking spray

Salt and freshly ground black pepper to taste

Dill sprigs and lime slices, for serving

Marinade

½ cup chopped fresh thyme

½ cup chopped fresh dill

½ cup chopped fresh rosemary

2 medium limes, juiced

1 tablespoon olive oil

*P*repare the marinade the night before the fish is to be cooked. The fish should marinate in the fridge overnight in a tightly covered or wrapped dish. To prepare the marinade, wash and chop the herbs, then mix with lime juice and 1 tablespoon olive oil.

Wash and drain the snapper fillets and place in the marinade, making sure the marinade is spooned over the fish on both sides several times. Cover tightly and let set overnight in the fridge.

The next day, sauté the bell peppers, onions, and garlic in 1 tablespoon olive oil, then set aside. Generously spray a nonstick grill pan with olive oil cooking spray and heat. Add the snapper fillets to the hot pan, season with salt and pepper to taste, and grill on both sides until browned. Turn with a nonstick spatula. Add the sautéed peppers and onions to reheat on top of the fish and serve with sprigs of dill and lime slices. Serves 4.

Nutritional Analysis: *calories: 190, protein: 32.4 grams, carbohydrate: 6.9 grams, fat: 3.7 grams, saturated fat: 0.8 grams, vitamin A: 1,635 IU, vitamin C: 130 milligrams, dietary fiber: 1.6 grams* ■

Dr. Ro's Country-City Cabbage

½ pound smoked turkey necks

1 small head of green cabbage, quartered

½ cup chopped fresh dill, or ½ cup dried dill

½ teaspoon minced garlic

1 small onion, peeled and quartered

1 teaspoon seasoned salt

*I*n a medium stockpot, bring 3 cups of water to a boil over high heat. Reduce the heat and boil the smoked turkey necks for approximately 1 hour, or until tender. Add the cabbage, dill, garlic, onion, and seasoned salt. Simmer for about 20 minutes, or until the cabbage is tender but firm and bright green. Serves 4.

Nutritional Analysis: *calories: 111, protein: 12.5 grams, carbohydrate: 9.5 grams, fat: 3.2 grams, saturated fat: 1 gram, cholesterol: 46 milligrams, vitamin C: 50 milligrams, dietary fiber: 3.7 grams* ■

Dr. Ro's New-Soul Mac-n-Cheese

2 tablespoons reduced-fat, trans-fat-free soft tub margarine

1 11½-ounce package elbow macaroni (whole-wheat noodles)

Salt (optional)

White pepper to taste

1 8-ounce package reduced-fat Cheddar cheese, shredded

5 cups skim milk

½ cup finely chopped softened sun-dried tomatoes

Paprika

*P*reheat the oven to 350°F.
Melt the margarine in a 2-quart casserole dish. Add the dry pasta and stir to coat with the margarine. Add the salt, if using, and pepper. Mix together half of the cheese, the milk, ¼ cup water, and the tomatoes. Pour over the macaroni. Reserve a small amount of the shredded cheese. Add the remaining ingredients with ¼ cup water and mix well. Sprinkle the reserved cheese over the top of the macaroni and cheese dish. Sprinkle with a hint of

paprika ('cause you wouldn't be black if you didn't). Bake for 1 to 1½ hours, until the liquid is fully absorbed. Serves 10.

Nutritional Analysis: *calories: 239, cholesterol: 7 milligrams (may vary according to your brand of cheese), fat: 3.4 grams (may also vary according to cheese), sodium: approx. 300 mg* ■

Dr. Ro's Country Steamed Apples
with a Twist

3 medium Granny Smith apples

2 medium McIntosh apples

¼ teaspoon ground cinnamon

⅛ teaspoon grated nutmeg

2 tablespoons brown sugar or 2 teaspoons sugar substitute (optional)

*C*ut the apples into small pieces. Place the apple pieces into a nonstick pan with the spices, sugar, and ¼ cup water. Cover and simmer until the apples become softened, gradually adding more water if necessary. Stir frequently to prevent the apples from sticking to the pan.

After cooking approximately 10 minutes, the apples should be soft and firm, not mushy, and should have a sweet and tart taste. Serves 4.

Nutritional Analysis: *calories: 187, fat: 0.576 grams, saturated fat: 0.95 grams, cholesterol: 0 milligrams, dietary fiber: 8.7 grams, vi-*

tamin A: 11.91 IU, vitamin C: 72 milligrams, calcium: 47.63 milligrams, iron: 1.91 milligrams ■

Dr. Ro's Steamed
Rainbow Potatoes and Onions

6 medium potatoes
  (a combination of new red,
  Yukon gold, and purple)
2 small onions
  (1 each yellow and red)

2 tablespoons olive oil
2 tablespoons minced garlic
Crushed red pepper to taste

*C*ut the potatoes into small cubes. Cut the onions into small slivers. Brown the potatoes and onions in a nonstick pan with olive oil. Add the garlic and crushed red pepper as the potatoes become brown and the onions become soft and opaque. Add ½ cup water and cover the pan tightly. Stir frequently to prevent the vegetables from sticking to the pan. The potato and onion mixture is done when the potatoes are brown and firm, yet soft, and the onions are limp. Serves 4.

Nutritional Analysis: *calories: 297, protein: 5.4 grams, fat: 7.2 grams, saturated fat: 1 gram, cholesterol: 0 milligrams, vitamin A: 187 IU, vitamin C: 36 milligrams, calcium: 36 milligrams, iron: 1 milligram* ■

Dr. Ro's Seafood-Tofu Stir-Fry

2 tablespoons sesame
  or peanut oil

1 cup broccoli florets

1 cup cauliflower florets

1 cup carrots, sliced
  on an angle

1 cup asparagus, sliced
  on an angle

½ cup water chestnuts

½ cup celery, sliced
  on an angle

2 spring onions, chopped,
  with green tops

½ pound scallops

½ pound medium shrimp,
  shelled and deveined, with
  tails

6 ounces firm tofu, cubed

Steamed brown rice or
  whole-wheat noodles,
  for serving

Stir-Fry Sauce

2 tablespoons crushed ginger

2 teaspoons crushed garlic

2 tablespoons low-sodium
  soy sauce

4 tablespoons fat-free
  vegetable broth

3 tablespoons rice wine
  (optional)

1 teaspoon sugar substitute
  (optional)

*B*lend the sauce ingredients in a mixing bowl with a wire whisk until smooth. Heat a wok or large nonstick skillet over high heat. Add the oil. Add the vegetables and stir-fry until nearly tender, about 2 minutes. Add the seafood and tofu, then the sauce and mix. Toss until the vegetables, seafood, and tofu are tender but firm. Serve over steamed brown rice or whole-wheat noodles. Serves 4.

Nutritional Analysis: *calories: 165, protein: 11.8 grams, carbohydrate: 8.5 grams, fat: 9.7 grams, saturated fat: 1.4 grams, cholesterol: 43 milligrams, vitamin C: 50 milligrams, vitamin A: 3,368 IU, dietary fiber: 1.9 grams* ∎

Dr. Ro's N'Awlins Butter Beans with Chicken Andouille Sausage

1 16-ounce can large butter beans

1 10-ounce can whole tomatoes

4 carrots, shredded

1 small onion, peeled and cubed

½ cup chopped fresh thyme

1 tablespoon crushed garlic

Salt and freshly ground black pepper to taste

3 chicken andouille sausage links, sliced on an angle

In a medium stockpot, bring the beans, tomatoes, carrots, onion, thyme, garlic, salt and pepper, and sausage to a boil. Reduce the heat and simmer for 30 minutes, or until the beans are tender and the sausage has shrunk to small disks. Serve hot with Dr. Ro's Corny Bread. Serves 4 to 6.

Nutritional Analysis: *calories: 175, protein: 12 grams, carbohydrate: 27.9 grams, fat: 5.3 grams, saturated fat: 0.9 grams, vitamin A: 17,390 IU, vitamin C: 17 milligrams, dietary fiber: 7.5 grams* ■

Dr. Ro's Corny Bread

½ cup canola oil

1½ cups yellow cornmeal

1½ cups whole-wheat flour

½ instant powdered
    nonfat milk

½ teaspoon salt

1½ teaspoons baking powder

3 tablespoons sugar (optional)

½ cup whole kernel corn

3 large egg whites

1½ cups skim milk

*P*reheat the oven to 400°F. Pour 1 tablespoon oil into an 8x8-inch square baking dish and grease the pan. Set aside. In a bowl, mix cornmeal, flour, powdered milk, salt, baking powder, and sugar, if using. Fold in the corn and set aside. In another bowl, beat the egg whites with a wire whisk until slightly frothy. Add the milk and remaining oil, and whisk again. Pour the liquid ingredients into the dry ingredients and mix. The remaining lumps are supposed to be there. Place the baking dish in the oven for 3 to 4 minutes to heat the oil. Don't burn it! Pour the batter into the baking dish and bake for approximately 20 minutes, or until golden brown. Corny Bread is done when a knife goes into its center and comes out clean. Remove from the oven immediately when done and turn the bread over on a cutting board. Cut into 12 squares and serve corn bread like your mama made, with a twist. *SAVOR THE FLAVOR! Serves 12.*

Nutritional Analysis: *calories: 185, fat: 5.1 grams, cholesterol: 1 milligram, sodium: 236 milligrams* ■

Kick-Start Your Way to
Livin' Healthy with Fitness

If you need a reason to get moving, try these on for size: weight loss, a boost to your immune system, stress relief, and a reduction in your risk of the chronic diseases you've read about in every chapter of this book: obesity, heart disease, diabetes, hypertension, and stroke. Did you know that regular exercise decreases both your systolic and diastolic blood pressure by 10 points, and that you can see this effect within three to four weeks of increasing your activity level? There is a mountain of good reasons to get fit, and by now you may be on board for making the commitment. But how will you go about changing your life for the better? It's as simple as putting one foot before the other.

This Life Was Made for Walking

I've said it many times: When you want to be healthy and you've exhausted all of your options, take a hike! If you truly are serious about wanting to improve the quality of your life, and I believe you are, then think about the good news. Walking as a form of physical fitness and exercise can lower your cholesterol level; reduce your risk of heart attack, osteoporosis, and breast and colon cancer; reduce constipation; lessen depression; flatten your tummy; tighten your

Calorie Payoff for Your Walk

If you weigh 120 pounds, you burn 80 calories per mile.

If you weigh 150 pounds, you burn 100 calories per mile.

If you weigh 180 pounds, you burn 115 calories per mile.

If you weigh 200 pounds, you burn 125 calories per mile.

thighs; and make you feel good about yourself. I know it sounds like a miracle. It isn't, but it's the next best thing to really getting you to the zone you want to live in for the rest of your productive and healthy life.

Here's the Evidence

According to one study, a brisk walk is as effective as running in reducing the risk of heart attack and stroke. Researchers studied 74,000 women between 50 and 79 and found that walking briskly for 2½ hours a week cut their heart attack and stroke risk by one-third. You can even walk away from high blood pressure—scientists reported that regular physical activity, such as brisk walking for 30 to 45 minutes five times a week, can reduce hypertension in people who already have it and could prevent its development in people who are susceptible to the disease. Other research shows that walking, combined with a healthful diet, is more effective in warding off diabetes than a popular drug.

The Nurses' Health Study, which I've referred to frequently throughout this book, found reductions in breast cancer risk among 122,000 participants who walked or exercised more vigorously at least seven hours per week, compared to women who exercised only one hour or less. Still not convinced that regular exercise is well worth your time?

Forgot where you put your keys lately? Or maybe you've dialed a number and forgotten who you called? What would you say if I told you that a study has shown that older women who walk regularly are less likely to develop memory loss compared to less active women? Another study showed that a brisk 30-minute walk or jog around a track three times a week was as effective as antidepressant medication in treating symptoms of depression. Imagine that. Walking protects bone density in the hips, too. A number of credible studies have been done showing that walking and life-long exercise protect bone density in the spine. And what about your cholesterol level? Had that checked lately? One study showed that women ages 74 to 87 who walked three days a week for 10 weeks significantly increased their HDL (good) cholesterol. Other studies have shown that moderate exercise decreases LDL (bad) cholesterol levels. So what have you got to lose except a shot at the good life?

Gearing Up to Get Started

So what gear will you need to get yourself on the road to healthy livin'? First, you'll need to invest in a pair of good walking shoes. If you cover 10 miles a week, you may need to replace them after a year. Your clothes should be comfortable and breathable and should not limit your steps or movement. Focus on getting out to walk, not on how you look. Once you reach a goal, you may want to reward yourself by buying a piece of fitness gear as a motivational tool.

How to Walk

Start your walking program slowly. The main goal at this point is to do it and stick with it. You may fall off the wagon from time to time, but remember, it's not how you start, it's how you end up. So each day is a new opportunity to get it right. That's what you must keep telling yourself. This is not a contest; it is not a get-slim-quick scheme. It is a lifestyle, and you must take it—but not yourself—seriously. Laugh on those days when you've done or said something truly crazy in an attempt to talk yourself out of what you know you should do. Don't beat yourself up, but do self-talk like "You can do it" and "Get out there," even when it's hard. Whatever you do, keep on pushing. This is the time when you must tell yourself, no matter how hard it is, "I've got to do this for me." Don't allow the kids, the job, the duties at the church, or your man to get in the way. Instead, take all of them with you. Take the family with you to make it a family affair. Take the church with you to make your church home one that's livin' for good health.

Begin by walking for 20 minutes a day if you haven't walked or done any kind of exercise recently. If you have, by all means challenge yourself and do more. Start by walking three days a week. After a few weeks, add another day. A few weeks later, move up to five days a week. A leisurely walk by some people's standards is better than no walk at all, but if you want to see real results, you must get to the point where you can barely hold a conversation while you're walking. This may not come at first, but trust me—it will come eventually. Set a goal of walking briskly enough to cover a mile in 15 minutes. At that rate you can burn as many calories as running that same mile in half the time. Take a look at the box on page 393 to see how many calories you burn by walking at various weight levels.

This Is How We Do It

* Be sure to keep your back straight and your head up.
* Keep your arms swinging at your sides (keep 'em movin').
* Don't walk flat-footed; instead, land on your heels and roll forward onto the balls of your feet.
* Keep breathing deeply and rhythmically with each step.
* To step it up, increase your steps rather than your stride. This reduces injuries.
* Warm up for at least five minutes, then stretch all of your muscle groups. Hold each stretch for 30 beats.

Who's Gonna Take the Weight?

If you are 35 or older, you should be thinking about adding weights to your workout. This is necessary to prepare for the bone mass that you'll lose as a result of menopause. I recommend that even younger women add weights to their workouts, because training with weights helps you build muscle and therefore burn fat more efficiently. Remember, the greater your muscle to fat ratio, the more fat you burn, even at rest. Weight training builds strong muscles and bones and helps you to obtain a trimmer, fitter body. You will become more fit if you add strength training to your routine after your daily walk. All it takes is an additional half hour. This should result in a total of one hour a day for your workout. Do that five days a week, eat according to my Color Plate System, then watch the results. They won't come overnight, but they will come.

Start Your Own Dr. Ro's Livin' Healthy Club

As part of your new commitment to livin' well, I challenge you to take charge of your life and put this plan into action. How? By starting your own Livin' Healthy Club.

All you need is a friend, family member, neighbor, church member, or classmate and a commitment to stay true to yourself. You can do this club with as few as two members, but the challenge will be more fruitful if there are more members. There is no formal structure, such as officers, unless you prefer to organize your club in that way. The purpose of the Livin' Healthy Club is to get some structure to your life and develop a support system for your new commitment and lifestyle. You will follow the diet and the exercise plan that you developed to fit your needs using the guidelines in this book. Grab the hands of some partners and sign them up for the Livin' Healthy Club. The club should go on walks together and share recipes, meals, triumphs, pitfalls, and challenges. The club should meet regularly to discuss lifestyle, share how you're managing your own, and trade insights on how the lessons you learned might benefit others. It would be very easy to blow this opportunity off and continue to sit on the couch and make excuses about why you're not livin' to your full potential. It is work to do otherwise. One study of almost 3,000 women found that the reasons most women give for not working out are family, lack of time, and lack of energy. You are the caregiver, but in your efforts to take care of everyone else, you have neglected yourself for too long. Isn't it time you changed your mind in order to change your life? Try it and let me know how it works for you. I know it will if you just give it a chance. Get some life. Life is for the livin'!

Acknowledgments

Gratitude Knows No Bounds

The first secret I learned, and the most valuable of my life lessons, came from my mother, Larvenia L. Brock, and my guardian, Rosetta H. Lewis. It was that I am valued and invaluable. All that I am and all that I will become are due to the sense of self-worth these two women gave me. Once I had that, it was natural for growth and maturity to teach me that a sense of self-worth imposes the responsibility of taking good care of that self. And because I value me, I also place a high value on all other human spirits and wish to share what I know with others. Many of the following beautiful, thoughtful, talented, and generous spirits contributed, directly or indirectly, to helping me do that in this work.

To Aunt Thelma and Uncle Frank, who shared in my rearing and who gave of themselves as if they had brought me into this world, a sincere thank-you for being there for me all these years.

To Dr. Murray Joseph Riggins Jr., a healer, a partner, and my most compassionate, supportive, and loving husband

and friend, thank you for being keenly aware of the complexities of the human spirit and of human nature and teaching me to embrace them to be better.

To my editor, Beth Rashbaum, whose dedication to leaving no stone unturned, no *t*'s uncrossed, and no *i*'s undotted gave this work depth and meaning, thank you for your intellect, skill, and mission for your craft. Your support is a constant reminder that there is good work to be done and that together we are stewards in this process to bring it to fruition. To Virginia Norey, a heartfelt thanks for your beautiful and culturally sensitive design for this book.

To my agent and friend, Barbara Lowenstein, who gets the deal done, thank you for your friendship, your support, and your belief in me. Books are business but you make the business of writing a healthy and inspiring process.

To Kendra Lee (my *Heart & Soul* editor), who reads everything I write before it goes anywhere, thank you for your sistahood, your patience, and your quiet-storm convictions. You are my shero, a true treasure to work with and to know.

To the women and their families whose stories appear in these pages, thank you for so generously sharing your experiences for the benefit of others.

To Dr. Allan A. Johnson, a mentor whom I proudly call a friend, your input was invaluable in getting the facts straight and helping me deliver an accurate manuscript. When I was a graduate student you taught me to challenge myself, and you continue to challenge me even today. To Dr. Barbara F. Harland, a friend and a minerals wiz, thanks for your careful review and critique of the material and for your thoughtful insight. To the other members of the nutrition faculty at Howard University, thanks for your brilliance, for your dedication to the field, and for helping me to use what I know to improve the lifestyle quality of the collective.

To Dawanna James, a gentle spirit and much-needed addition to the nutrition profession, a heartfelt thanks for all the research you did to help me get my facts and figures right.

To Deborah C. Tang, thanks for giving me my first break on Black Entertainment Television. You changed my life!

To Pearline and John Singletary, my new parents, thank you for your unyielding love and support.

To the fans of *Heart & Soul* TV and of Dr. Ro, many thanks for the years of support and for the questions and input (solicited and unsolicited) that served to further my growth and expertise. Without you, this work would have no place.

To Patricia Smith, Ken Sanders, Petr, and the many trainers who so generously gave of themselves for my improvement, I am better and more fit for having known and been supported by you. To Ken, you are the man! Thank you for sculpting this body day after tireless day. Because of you I have finally grown to accept my lot in life—to work out or get out of the business!

To Alana Alexander, a graduate student among grad students, thank you for your tireless dedication and your unyielding support in this work. You stepped up to the plate at the time I most needed help.

To Denise Hinds of Uzuri Braids, a heartfelt thanks for twisting my tresses for the book jacket and caring for my natural mane, always.

To my sista-friends who allow me to be me and who love me anyway, you know who you are, but here are a few names: the crab-leg crew (Mary Rullow, Drs. Kim Callwood, Bolivia Davis, and Shelly Hope DeMass,

Attorney Patricia Davis, Evelyn Minor), my sistas Cheryl Quick and Gloria Wiggs, and Renee Booker. Thanks for your love and support. To my *Heart & Soul* co-host and sista-friend, Mocha Lee, thanks for being my fitness muse. Like the book says, sitting next to you was motivation enough to put down the steak and cheese sub and get my butt off the couch!

Peace, blessings, and always good health to you all!

Notes

Secret ☆

Battling Denial

Page 24: "The report estimates that a staggering 61 percent of American adults"

Satcher, David (2001) "The Surgeon General's Call to Action to Prevent and Decrease Overweight and Obesity." Washington, D.C.: U.S. Department of Health and Human Services, Public Health Service, Office of the Surgeon General, Rockville, Maryland.

Page 29: "at 20 pounds more than their healthy weight"

Rand, C. S. W. and Kuldau, J. M. (1990) "The epidemiology of obesity and self-defined weight problems in the general population: Gender, race, age, and social class." *International Journal of Eating Disorders:* 329–343.

Secret 2

Good News: Bone mass statistics

Page 44: "black women have greater bone mass"

Ellis, Ken, Director of the Body Composition Laboratory at Baylor College of Medicine, Houston, Texas (2000) "Ask *Heart & Soul.*" *Heart & Soul Magazine*, October/November 2000.

Ortiz, O., Russell, M., Daley, T. L., Baumgartner, R. N., Waki, M., Lichtman, S., Wang, J., Pierson, R.N., Heymsfield, S. (1992) "Differences in skeletal muscle and bone mineral mass between black and white females and their relevance to estimates of body composition." *American Journal of Clinical Nutrition* 55: 8–13.

Bad News: African American's predisposition to obesity: Thrifty gene

Page 44: "a gene called the thrifty gene"

American Heart Association News Release: (November 13, 2000) "High blood pressure gene also linked to obesity."

Personal Interview with Dr. Francine Kaufman, pediatric endocrinologist and noted obesity and type II diabetes researcher of the National Institutes of Health.

Page 45: "obese black sistas burn 33 fewer calories . . . than their white sisters"

Christian, W., Soren, S., Borgardus, C., and Ravussin, E. (1999) "Energy metabolism in African Americans: potential risk factors for obesity." *Journal of Clinical Nutrition* 70: 13–20.

Weinsier, R. L., Hunter, G. R., et al. (2000) "Energy expenditure and free-living physical activity in black and white women: comparison before and after weight loss." *Journal of Clinical Nutrition* 71: 1138–1146.

Forman, J. N., Miller, W. C., Szymanski, L. M., and Fernhall, B. (1998) "Differences in resting metabolism rates of inactive obese African American and Caucasian women." *Obesity* 22: 215–221.

Pages 46–47: "over one in two black women age 40 and over is obese" Centers for Disease Control and Prevention, www.cdc.org.

Flefal, K. W., Carroll, M.D., Ogden, C. L., and Johnson, C. L. (2002) "Prevalence and trends in obesity among U.S. adults, 1999–2000." *Journal of the American Medical Association* 288: 1723–1732.

Heart Disease

Page 49: "the death rate from CHD among black women"

Mosca, L., Manson, J. A. E., Sutherland, S. E., Langer, R. D., Manolito, R., Barrett-Connor, E. (1997) "Cardiovascular disease in women: A statement for healthcare professionals from the American Heart Association." *Circulation* 96: 2468–2482.

Reaven, Gerald, M.D., Strom, Terry Kristen, M.B.A., and Fox, Barry, Ph.D. (2000) *Syndrome X: Overcoming the Silent Killer That Can Give You a Heart Attack* (New York: Simon and Schuster).

Report of the Scientific Sessions (November 13, 2000). The American Heart Association Scientific Sessions, New Orleans, LA.

Blacks and sodium retention due to middle passage

Page 51: "because those slaves whose bodies could hold on to salt were more likely to survive"

"Study identifies hypertension patients who can benefit from the little used diuretic amiloride: An intriguing hypothesis surmises that higher incidence of hypertension in African Americans may be related to slave ship crossings." American Physiological Society (APS) press release from August 19, 2002.

"Body's appetite suppressant linked to high blood pressure in African Americans." Press release, Medical College of Wisconsin Cardiovascular Center, August 1999.

Singleton, L., Johnson, K., Villarosa, L. (1993) *The Black Health Library Guide to Stroke* (New York: Henry Holt and Co.).

Blacks and stress-related hypertension

Pages 51–52: "African Americans . . . suffer unusually high levels of stress"

Krieger, N. and Sidney, S. (1996) "Racial discrimination and blood pressure: the CARDIA Study of young black and white adults." *American Journal of Public Health* 86: 1370–1378.

Harrell, J. P. (1980), "Psychological factors and hypertension: a status report." *Psychological Bulletin* 87: 482–501.

Harrell, J. P., Hall, S., and Taliaferro, J. (2003) "Physiological responses to racism and discrimination: an assessment of the evidence." *American Journal of Public Health* 93: 243–248.

Daniels, I. N., Harrell, J. P., Floyd, L. J., and Bell, S. R. (2001) "Hostility, cultural orientation, and casual blood pressure readings in African Americans." *Ethnic Diseases* 11: 779–787.

Jones, D. R., Harrell, J. P., Morris-Prather, C. E., Thomas, J., and Omowale, N. (1996) "Affective and physiological responses to racism: the role of afrocentrism and mode of presentation." *Ethnic Diseases* 6: 109–122.

Cardillo, C., Cresence, K. M., Cannon, R. O., and Panza, J. O. (1998) "Racial differences in nitric oxide-mediated vasodilator response to mental stress in the forearm circulation." *Hypertension* 31: 1235–1239.

"Study reveals possible clue for racial differences in prevalence of high blood pressure." American Heart Association press release, June 18, 1999.

Clark, R., Anderson, N. B., Clark, V. R., Williams, D. R. (1999) "Racism as a stressor for African Americans: A biopsychosocial model." *American Psychologist* 54: 805–816.

"Study: Racist provocation triggers potentially damaging physical, emotional symptoms." Press release, Duke Medical Center, July 15, 1996.

Page 52: "a sedentary lifestyle accounts for 12 percent of hypertension cases"

Centers for Disease Control and Prevention (February 2003)."The promise of prevention, reducing the health and economic burden of chronic disease." Department of Health and Human Services, Centers for Disease Control and Prevention.

Breast Cancer

Page 55: "African American women are more likely to die"

"Cancer health disparities." Fact sheet, National Cancer Institute website, www.cancer.gov.

Page 55: "risk is increased . . . if she gains belly fat"

Nagi, K. B., Cantor, A., Allen, K., et al. (2000) "Android obesity at diagnosis and breast carcinoma survival." *Cancer* 88: 2751–2757.

Apple-shaped women and increased risk for breast cancer

Page 55: "apple-shaped women were 34 percent more likely to develop breast cancer"

Huang, Z., Willet, W. C., Colditz, G. A., Hunter, D. J., Manson, J. E., Rosner, B., Speizer, F. E., and Hankinson, S. E. (1999), "Waist circumference, waist, hip ratio, and risk of breast cancer in the Nurses' Health Study." *American Journal of Epidemiology* 150: 1316–1324.

African Americans and Hispanic Americans (Mexican Americans) and metabolic syndrome

Page 63: "African American people and Hispanic people appear more likely to have metabolic syndrome"

Ford, E. S., Giles, W. H., and Dietz, W. H. (2002) "Prevalence of the metabolic syndrome among U.S. adults: findings from the Third National Health and Examination Survey." *Journal of the American Medical Association* 287: 356–359.

Stress and weight gain in the belly region

Page 70: "looked at 59 premenopausal women"

Epel, E. S., McEwen, B., Castellazzo, G., Brownell, K. D., Bell, J., and Ickovics, J. R. (2000) "Stress and body shape: stress-induced cortisol secretion among women with central fat." *Psychosomatic Medicine* 62: 623–632.

Fifteen-minute exercise bouts to reduce heart disease risk

Page 78: "two 15-minute aerobic exercise sessions can curb heart disease risk"

I-Min, L., Sesso, H. D., Paffenbarger, R. S., Jr. (2000) "Physical activity and coronary heart disease in men." *Circulation* 102: 981.

Secret ✪

Beans, Beans, Good for (More than) Your Heart

Page 96: "isoflavones in soybeans...play a key role... keeps your arteries supple"

Van der Schouw, Y. T., Pijpe, A., Lebrun, C. E. I, et al. (2002) "Higher usual dietary intake of phytoestrogens is associated with lower aortic stiffness in postmenopausal women." *Arteriosclerosis, Thrombosis, and Vascular Biology* 22: 1316.

Pages 96–97: "women who ate these legumes...had a 22 percent lower risk"

Bazzano, L. A., Jiang, H. E., Ogden, L. G., Loria, C., et al. (2001) "Legume consumption and risk of coronary heart disease in U.S. men and women." *Archives of Internal Medicine* 161: 2573.

Page 100: "nurses who ate the most sugars and refined carbohydrates"

Salmeron, J., Manson, J. E., et al. (1997) "Dietary fiber, glycemic load, and risk of non-insulin-dependent diabetes mellitus in women." *Journal of the American Medical Association* 277: 472.

Page 102: "women who eat three servings of whole grains a day have half the risk"

Simin, L., Stampfer, M. J., et al. (1999) "Whole-grain consumption and risk of coronary heart disease: results from the Nurses' Health Study." *American Journal of Clinical Nutrition* 70: 412–419.

Page 105: "ellagic acid seems to trigger a process called apoptosis"

Narayanan, B. A., Geoffroy, O. Willingham, M. C., Nixon, D. W. (1999) "p53/p21(WAF1/C1P1) expression and its possible role in G1 arrest and apoptosis in ellagic acid treated cancer cells." *Cancer Letters* 136: 215–221.

Pages 106–107: "hormones . . . may contribute to fibroids"

Lark, Susan. *Fibroid Tumors & Endometriosis.* (Berkeley: Self-Help Book: Celestial Arts.)

Milloy, Marilyn (2000). "Calming fibroids–naturally." *Heart & Soul Magazine*, April/May: 60–61.

"Prevent fibroids with a color shift." (2000) *Prevention* magazine, February: 36.

Television news interview, BET News, Black Entertainment Television, Dr. Rovenia Brock, medical correspondent, 2002.

Television interview, *Heart & Soul*, Black Entertainment Television, Dr. Rovenia Brock, host/medical correspondent, 2001.

Page 110: "Two major studies . . . found that"

Rossouw, J. E. et al. (2002) "Risks and benefits of estrogen plus progestin in healthy postmenopausal women: Principal results from the Women's Health Initiative randomized controlled trial." *Journal of the American Medical Association* 288: 321–333.

Lacey, J. V., Mink, P. J., et al. (2002) "Menopausal hormone replacement therapy and risk of ovarian cancer." *Journal of the American Medical Association* 288: 334–341.

Secret 5

How we got where we are today: The advice that backfired

Page 167: "they found a general trend toward lower blood pressure levels in people who consumed more . . . high calcium foods"

Freudenheim, J. L., Russell, M., Trevisan, M., and Doemland, M. (1991) "Calcium intake and blood pressure in blacks and whites." *Ethnic Diseases* 1: 114–122.

Pages 177–178: "a recent study found that older women . . . burned calories just as fast as younger women"

Melanson, K. J., Saltzman, E., Russell, R. R., and Roberts, S. B. (1997) "Fat oxidation in response to four graded energy challenges in younger and older women." *American Journal of Clinical Nutrition* 66: 860–866.

Page 183: "Gary Taubes wrote an article"

Taubes, G. (2002) "What If It's All Been a Big Fat Lie?" *New York Times Magazine*, July 7: 22.

Secret ⚙

Fast food in the nation's hospitals

Pages 189–190: "a third of the nation's top hospitals now have fast-food franchises in their cafeterias"

"Fast-food franchises in hospitals." (2002) Letter to the editor, *Journal of the American Medical Association*: 287.

Antioxidants in black tea

Page 204: "a serving of black tea had more antioxidants"

Prior, R. L., and Cao, G. (1999) "Antioxidant capacity and polyphenolic components of teas: implications for altering in vivo antioxidant status." *Experimental Biology and Medicine* 220: 255–261.

Rice-Evans, C. (1999) "Implications of the mechanisms of action of tea polyphenols as antioxidants in vitro for chemoprevention in humans." *Proceedings Social and Experimental Biology and Medicine* 220: 262–266.

Secret 7

Childhood obesity

Page 224: "children . . . with a television in the bedroom"

Dennison, B. A., Erb, T. A., and Jenkins, P. L. (2002) "Television viewing and television in bedroom associated with overweight risk among low-income preschool children." *Pediatrics* 109: 1028–1035.

Page 224: "the rate of obesity increases 2 percent for each hour of TV"

Dietz, W. H., Jr., Gortmaker, S. L. (1985) "Do we fatten our children at the television set? Obesity and television viewing in children and adolescents." *Pediatrics* 75: 807–812.

"Television and obesity among children." Fact sheet, National Institute on Media and the Family. www.media andthefamily.org.

Page 226: "Fat kids will more than likely become fat adults"

Whitaker, R. C., Deeks, C. M., Baughcum, A. E., and Specker, B. L. (2000) "The relationship of childhood adiposity to parent body mass index and eating behavior." *Obesity Research* 8: 234–240.

Guo, S. S., Wu, W., Chumlea, W. C., and Roche, A. F. (2002) "Predicting overweight and obesity in adulthood from body mass index values in childhood and adolescence." *American Journal of Clinical Nutrition* 76: 497–498.

Shumei, S., Guo, S. S., and Chumlei, W. C. (1999) "Tracking of body mass index in children in relation to overweight in adulthood." *American Journal of Clinical Nutrition* 70: 145s–148s.

Page 226: "fatty streaks had already begun to form"

Berenson, G. S., Wattigney, W. A., Tracy, R. E., Newman, W. P., Srinivassan, S. R., Webber, L. S., Dalferes, E. R., Strong, J. P. (1992) "Atherosclerosis of the aorta and coronary arteries and cardiovascular risk factors in persons aged 6 to 30 years and studied at necropsy (The Bogalusa Heart Study)." *American Journal of Cardiology* 70: 851–858.

The Bogalusa Heart Study Autopsy, the Bogalusa Heart Study website: www.som.tulane.edu (Tulane University).

Page 227: "as many as 45 percent of newly diagnosed cases of diabetes"

"Children and diabetes." American Diabetes Association fact sheet. www. diabetes.org.

Page 227: "25 percent had impaired glucose tolerance"

Ranjana, S., Fisch, G., et al. (2002) "Prevalence of impaired glucose tolerance among children and adolescents with marked obesity." *New Journal of Medicine* 346: 22.

Page 231: "the link between obesity and early maturation may be related to the hormone leptin"

Lemonick, M. D. (2000) "Teens Before Their Time." *Time* magazine: October 30.

Page 244: "the amount of regular exercise girls get falls off dramatically"

Kimm, S. Y. S, Glynn, N. W., Krisha, A. M., et al. (2002) "Decline in physical activity in black girls and white girls during adolescence." *New England Journal of Medicine* 347: 709–715.

Page 256: "black girls tend to have better self-images"

Kumanyika, S. (1998) "Obesity in African Americans: Biobehavioral consequences of culture." *Ethnicity and Disease* 8: 93–96.

Kumanyika, S., Wilson, J. F., and Guilford-Davenport, M. (1993) "Weight-related attitudes and behaviors of black women." *Journal of the American Dietetic Association* 93: 416–422.

Dotson, V. "Body image in African American women." Vanderbilt University Department of Psychology, www.vanderbilt.edu/AnS/psychology/health_psychology/Vashti.htm.

Kumanyika, S., and Morssink, C. B. (1997) *Overweight and Weight Management*, Chapter 3: Cultural appropriateness of weight management programs." (Gaithersburg, MD: Aspen Publishers).

Secret ⚙

Page 285: "taking a multivitamin ... may reduce your risk of colon cancer"

Giovannucci, E., Stampfer, M. J., et al. (1998) "Multivitamin use, folate, and colon cancer in women in the Nurses' Health Study." *Annals of Internal Medicine* 29: 517–524.

Page 288: "Alpha-lipoic acid"

Heber, D., and Bowerman, S. (2001) *What Color Is Your Diet?* (New York: Regan Books).

Joseph, J. A., Nadeau, D. A., and Underwood, A. (2002) *The Color Code: A Revolutionary Eating Plan for Optimum Health* (New York: Hyperion).

Page 288: "Selenium"

Clark, L. C., Combs, G. F., et al. (1996) "Effects of selenium supplementation for cancer prevention in patients with carcinoma of the skin. A randomized controlled trial. Nutrition prevention of Cancer Study Group." *Journal of the American Medical Association* 276: 1957.

Page 289: "Pycnogenol"

Spadea, L., and Balestrazzi, E. (2001) "Treatment of vascular neuropathies with Pycnogenol." *Phytotherapy Research* 15: 219–223.

Page 289: "studies suggest that quercetin may also reduce coronary heart disease mortality rates and prevent diabetes"

Binsack, R., Boersma, B. J., et al. (2001) "Enhanced antioxidant activity after chlorination of quercetin by hypochlorous acid." *Alcohol: Clinical and Experimental Research* 25: 434–443.

Berkeley Wellness Letter, UC Berkeley (January, 2003). www.berkeleywellness.com.

Page 306: "Vitamin E . . . 400 to 800 IU of vitamin E has been shown to reduce heart attack risk."

Stephens, N. G., Parsons, A., et al. (1996) "Randomized controlled trial of vitamin E in patients with coronary heart disease: Cambridge Heart Antioxidant Study." *The Lancet* 347: 781–786.

Page 306: "people who took megadoses of vitamin E for five years suffered just as many strokes and heart attacks"

Salim, Y., Phil, D., Dagenais, G., et al. (2000) "Vitamin E supplementation and cardiovascular events in high-risk patients." *New England Journal of Medicine* 342: 154–160.

Secret 🐞

Page 311: "black folks have a 'poor quality' diet"

The Healthy Eating Index 1999–2000, USDA Publication.

Page 324: "those who ate nuts five times a week"

Jui, J., Manson, J. E., Meir, S. J., Simin, L., Willet, W. C., and Hu, F. B. (2002) "Nut and peanut butter consumption and risk of type 2 diabetes in women." *Journal of the American Medical Association* 288: 2554–2560.

Secret 🏅

Page 393: "a brisk walk is as effective as running"

Manson, J. E., Greenland, P., et al. (2002) "Walking compared with vigorous exercise for the prevention of cardiovascular events in women." *New England Journal of Medicine* 347: 716–725.

Page 393: "regular physical activity ... can reduce hypertension"

Whelton, S. P., Chin, A., Xue, X., and Jiang, H. (2002) "Effect of aerobic exercise on blood pressure: a meta-analysis of randomized, controlled trials." *Annals of Internal Medicine* 136: 493–503.

Page 394: "walking ... is more effective in warding off diabetes than a popular drug"

National Institutes of Health: National Institute of Diabetes and Digestive and Kidney Disorders website: www.niddk.nih.gov.

Breast cancer and exercise

Page 394: "reductions in breast cancer risk"

Rockhill, B., Willet, W. C., et al. (1999) "A prospective study of recreational physical activity and breast cancer risk" *Archives of Internal Medicine* 159: 2290–2296.

The benefits of walking

Page 394: "older women who walk regularly are less likely to develop memory loss"

Yaffe, K., Barnes, D., Nevitt, M., et al. (2001) "A prospective study of physical activity and cognitive decline in elderly women: women who walk." *Archives of Internal Medicine* 161: 1703–1708.

Page 394: "a brisk 30-minute walk...was as effective as antidepressant medication"

Blumenthal, J. A., Babyak, M. A., Moore, K. A., et al. (1999) "Effects of exercise training on older patients with major depression." *Archives of Internal Medicine* 159: 2349–2356.

Page 394: "women ages 74 to 87 who walked . . . significantly increased their HDL"

Fahlman, M. M., Boardley, D., Lambert, C., and Flynn, M. G. (2002) "Effects of endurance training and resistance training on plasma lipoprotein profiles in elderly women." *Journals of Gerontology* 57: B54–B60.

Resources

Nutrition

www.askdrro.com

The American Dietetic Association
National Center for Nutrition and Dietetics
216 West Jackson Boulevard
Chicago, Illinois 60606
Consumer Nutrition Hotline
(800) 366-1655
www.eatright.org

Cooperative Extension Service
Washington, D.C.
University of the District of Columbia
4200 Connecticut Avenue N.W.
Washington, D.C. 20008
(202) 274-7115
www.udc.edu

In other states: contact the local land-grant university

Food Allergy Network
10400 Eaton Place
Suite 107
Fairfax, Virginia 22030
(703) 691-3179

Food and Drug Administration (FDA)
Consumer Information Office
5600 Fishers Lane
HFE
Rockville, Maryland 20857
(301) 443-3170

Mayo Clinic Health Nutrition and Health Information
www.mayoclinic.com

Tufts University Diet and Nutrition Information
www.navigator.tufts.edu

United Fresh Fruit and Vegetable Association
(202) 303-3400

USDA Meat and Poultry Hotline
(800) 535-4555

Sports and Nutrition

Dr. Ro Gear
8639-B Sixteenth Street
Suite 193
Silver Spring, Maryland 20910
(877) 291-4240

In D.C. area
(202) 291-4240
www.drrogear.com
email: *drro@drrogear.com*

American College of Sports Medicine
P.O. Box 1440
Indianapolis, Indiana 46206
(317) 637-9200

American Council on Exercise
Consumer Fitness Hotline
(800) 529-8227

Health

[Cancer]
American Cancer Society
1599 Clifton Road, N.E.
Atlanta, Georgia 30329
(800) 227-2345
(404) 320-3333

National Cancer Institute
National Institutes of Health
31 Center Drive
Building 31- Room 10A07
Bethesda, Maryland 20892
(800) 4-cancer; (800) 422-6237

[Diabetes]
American Diabetes Association
1660 Duke Street
Alexandria, Virginia 22314
(800) 232-4372

National Diabetes Information Clearinghouse
2 Information Way
Bethesda, Maryland 20892
(301) 654-3327

[Heart Disease]
American Heart Association
7272 Greenville Avenue
Dallas, Texas 75231
(800) AHA-USA1; (800) 242-8721

National Cholesterol Education Program
National Heart, Lung and Blood Institute
P.O. Box 30105
Bethesda, Maryland 20824
(301) 251-1222

National Medical Association
1012 10th Street, N.W.
Washington, D.C. 20001
(202) 347-1895
www.nmanet.org

Index

About the Author

Rovenia M. Brock, Ph.D., has been a practicing nutritionist for over twenty years and was the host of Black Entertainment Television's *Heart & Soul*. An award-winning lecturer and health reporter, she is the resident nutrition expert to bet.com, where she writes the syndicated column, "Livin' Healthy with Dr. Ro," which also appears in newspapers. She is currently host of *Health Matters*, a health and lifestyles television program aired on WHUT, the Howard University PBS station. She lives in Washington, D.C., with her husband, Dr. Murray Riggins, and their beloved cocker spaniel, Destinye.